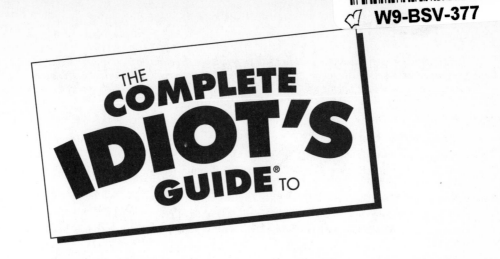

THE COMPLETE IDIOT'S GUIDE® TO

Gluten-Free Eating

by Eve Adamson and Tricia Thompson, MS, RD

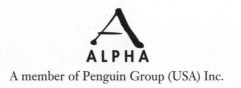

ALPHA

A member of Penguin Group (USA) Inc.

This book is for you, because you didn't ask to go gluten-free, but here you are. Remember what Shakespeare said: "Be not afraid of greatness. Some are born great, some achieve greatness, and others have greatness thrust upon them." May you finally find the great health you've been seeking.

ALPHA BOOKS

Published by the Penguin Group

Penguin Group (USA) Inc., 375 Hudson Street, New York, New York 10014, USA

Penguin Group (Canada), 90 Eglinton Avenue East, Suite 700, Toronto, Ontario M4P 2Y3, Canada (a division of Pearson Penguin Canada Inc.)

Penguin Books Ltd., 80 Strand, London WC2R 0RL, England

Penguin Ireland, 25 St. Stephen's Green, Dublin 2, Ireland (a division of Penguin Books Ltd.)

Penguin Group (Australia), 250 Camberwell Road, Camberwell, Victoria 3124, Australia (a division of Pearson Australia Group Pty. Ltd.)

Penguin Books India Pvt. Ltd., 11 Community Centre, Panchsheel Park, New Delhi—110 017, India

Penguin Group (NZ), 67 Apollo Drive, Rosedale, North Shore, Auckland 1311, New Zealand (a division of Pearson New Zealand Ltd.)

Penguin Books (South Africa) (Pty.) Ltd., 24 Sturdee Avenue, Rosebank, Johannesburg 2196, South Africa

Penguin Books Ltd., Registered Offices: 80 Strand, London WC2R 0RL, England

International Standard Book Number: 978-1-59257-683-8
Library of Congress Catalog Card Number: 2007928982

09   8   7   6   5

Interpretation of the printing code: The rightmost number of the first series of numbers is the year of the book's printing; the rightmost number of the second series of numbers is the number of the book's printing. For example, a printing code of 07-1 shows that the first printing occurred in 2007.

Printed in the United States of America

Note: This publication contains the opinions and ideas of its authors. It is intended to provide helpful and informative material on the subject matter covered. It is sold with the understanding that the authors, book producer, and publisher are not engaged in rendering professional services in the book. If the reader requires personal assistance or advice, a competent professional should be consulted.

The authors, book producer, and publisher specifically disclaim any responsibility for any liability, loss, or risk, personal or otherwise, which is incurred as a consequence, directly or indirectly, of the use and application of any of the contents of this book.

Most Alpha books are available at special quantity discounts for bulk purchases for sales promotions, premiums, fund-raising, or educational use. Special books, or book excerpts, can also be created to fit specific needs.

For details, write: Special Markets, Alpha Books, 375 Hudson Street, New York, NY 10014.

Publisher: *Marie Butler-Knight*
Editorial Director: *Mike Sanders*
Managing Editor: *Billy Fields*
Executive Editor: *Randy Ladenheim-Gil*
Book Producer: *Lee Ann Chearney/Amaranth Illuminare*
Development Editor: *Ginny Bess Munroe*
Production Editor: *Megan Douglass*

Copy Editor: *Nancy Wagner*
Cartoonist: *Steve Barr*
Cover Designer: *Bill Thomas*
Book Designer: *Trina Wurst*
Indexer: *Heather McNeill*
Layout: *Ayanna Lacey*
Proofreader: *John Etchison*

Contents at a Glance

Contents

Introduction

You've made the decision—or your body has made it for you. You'll live without gluten, no matter how difficult it is, because living *with* gluten has finally proven to be too great an obstacle. Whether you or someone you love has endured the stomachaches, the diarrhea, the gas, the joint pain, the headaches, or the fatigue; whether you've been misdiagnosed time and again (chronic fatigue syndrome? irritable bowel syndrome? any other syndrome?), or you just want to feel good for once in your life, you know now that giving up gluten will help set you on the right path.

But will you like it? Will you be able to stand it? Can you cook anything your gluten-intolerant child will eat? Can you go to your favorite restaurant? Will you ever enjoy eating food again if you can't have those warm rolls and steamy pasta and delicious cheesy pizzas? Perish the thought! Eating gluten-free can be a joy, a surprise, a great adventure, and the key to feeling better than you ever dreamed you could feel (and looking better, too!). This book is your key.

While we fill you in on everything you need to know, we don't spend a lot of time going into the technical stuff, the science, or the frankly unpleasant inner workings of gluten intolerance, although you can get the basics in Chapter 1. We know what you *really* want from a book like this—you want to know that you can go into your kitchen or out to a restaurant and find something delicious and satisfying to eat … something that won't make you sick, but that still satisfies your hunger. You want to know how to cook your favorite meals again, but without gluten. You want to know how to *live*.

This book gets right down to gluten-free nitty-gritty: what you can and can't eat and how to manage your life in a way that works, from cooking for your family to dining out to navigating food labels in the grocery store. You don't want your "special diet," or your child's special diet, to consume every waking moment; you just want to live your life and feel good. It's true—eating gluten-free can be a challenge, but that doesn't mean it has to be a chore.

So get ready to feel better, almost immediately. Get ready for your body to heal. Get ready for your child to regain glowing health. Get ready for your family to thrive. Get ready for your body to thank you with more energy, more vitality, and more life. And get ready to enjoy your food again. That's what eating gluten-free is all about.

About This Book

The Complete Idiot's Guide to Gluten-Free Eating is divided into five parts that break down gluten-free eating into manageable categories.

In **Part 1, "Gluten-Free Eating 101,"** we introduce you to the whole concept, answering all your questions like "What is gluten?" and "Why can't some people eat it?" We explain the tests to ask your doctor about if you think you might be gluten-intolerant, and we also give you lots of support if you already know you are. In this part, you get an introduction to the foods you must avoid, and a few tantalizing hints about the wonderful foods that are A-OK for you.

In **Part 2, "What to Eat and What to Avoid,"** learn how to read a food label and decipher what's what when it comes to ferreting out the gluten. Find out more about hidden glutens and how to avoid them, and what manufacturers *must tell you.* You'll also find helpful lists of foods that are often or always gluten-free, and lists of foods that are often or always gluten-filled, to help guide you in your quest to fill your pantry and refrigerator with healthy food you can actually enjoy.

Part 3, "Convenience and Temptation," begins with a primer on packaged food, from canned soup to that jar of nuts. Find out what's gluten-free and what's probably not. Next, enjoy a chapter dedicated to gluten-free packaged foods, including our personal favorites. Finally, find out the truth about beer, wine, and spirits—what you can enjoy, and what to avoid. Finally, you'll get a pep talk on how to survive out there, in a world full of temptation. You can do it!

In **Part 4, "Gluten-Free Dining,"** you might feel like you're in gluten-free cooking school. Find out how to make substitutions for gluten-filled ingredients so you can still cook your favorite foods, get started with easy recipes, and find a week of gluten-free menus to set you on the right path to gluten-free eating.

Part 5, "Out and About: Gluten-Free and Loving It!" covers eating in restaurants, bringing along gluten-free food so you never get stuck starving and faced with gluten-only options, and finally, a lesson on nutrition and health, because eating gluten-free is only half the battle. The other half is all about building your own health back up into the most spectacular and glowing you it's possible to be.

Extras

Throughout each chapter in this book, you'll find four types of extra information, nicely bundled into little boxes for your reading pleasure. These add to your practical knowledge, inspire you, sympathize, or caution you. These boxes are also guaranteed to be 100 percent gluten-free!

> **Fearless Eater**
>
> In these boxes we give you stories about our own experiences going gluten-free, so you can get some insight into what could happen: what the waitress said, what product tasted fabulous, what happened when we tried to find gluten-free snacks on the road or actually got to order gluten-free pasta in a restaurant … stuff like that.

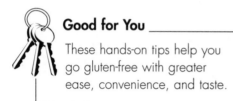

Good for You

These hands-on tips help you go gluten-free with greater ease, convenience, and taste.

def•i•ni•tion

We define unusual or specialized words in these boxes so you can be sure you know what the heck we are talking about.

Read the Label

These cautions are meant to be a heads-up for you about what to watch out for or be aware of as you live your gluten-free life.

Acknowledgments

Eve Adamson: Thanks to my kids for being so patient about this whole gluten-free thing. Okay, they really weren't all that patient, but they were willing to try recipes and products and were perfectly honest in letting me know which tasted great and which got the thumbs-down. (Let's just say I threw out a lot of homemade cookies …) Thanks also to Ben who always supports my dietary oddities and keeps me strong when I'm tempted to cheat. Thanks finally to Tricia, who made this whole gluten-free business seem much less complicated. She is a bright beacon in a dark, gluten-clogged world.

Tricia Thompson, MS, RD: A huge thank you to my husband Dave for his constant support and my son Marcus for being my inspiration. Neither of them ever make me feel that my eating gluten-free is an oddity—it is just the way things are. Thank you also to my colleague Joanne Larsen who in her very matter-of-fact way strongly encouraged me to take on this project. And finally thank you to Eve, whose refreshing writing style and willingness to "go gluten-free" truly make this book a unique contribution.

Trademarks

All terms mentioned in this book that are known to be or are suspected of being trademarks or service marks have been appropriately capitalized. Alpha Books and Penguin Group (USA) Inc. cannot attest to the accuracy of this information. Use of a term in this book should not be regarded as affecting the validity of any trademark or service mark.

Part 1

Gluten-Free Eating 101

In Part 1 of this book, you learn all the basics. What is gluten? Why shouldn't you eat it? How do you know if you're sensitive to it? What foods have it? Can you really *do* this, eat gluten-free? In this first part of the book, we answer all these questions and more. Whether you need a definition, want to know which foods and nonfood products have gluten, or really need some motivation to help you eat gluten-free successfully, you'll find it here.

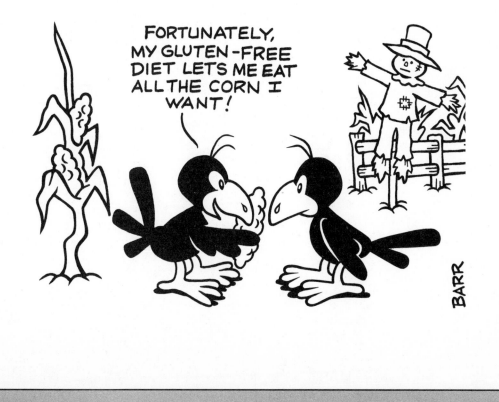

What's Wrong with Gluten?

In This Chapter

- ◆ Reasons I quit eating gluten
- ◆ Definition of gluten and its characteristics
- ◆ The symptoms of celiac disease and gluten intolerance
- ◆ Testing for celiac disease
- ◆ Working with your test results

It all started with a phone call: "Hi, Eve. It's Lee Ann. Do you want to write a book about gluten-free eating?"

"Do I want to write a book about what?"

When my gluten-free odyssey began, I—like many other people, including those who are diagnosed with celiac disease—didn't have the first idea what gluten was. Sure, I'd heard of it. It sounded unappealing, kind of glue-like and sticky (which, as a matter of fact, it is). But I didn't know what foods contained it, why I wouldn't want to eat it, or why my publishers would want me to write a book about it.

Back then, I didn't know that some people with celiac disease have a serious, dangerous autoimmune response to gluten. I didn't know that some people, even though they test negative for celiac disease, feel better when they stop eating gluten. And I certainly didn't know how the heck you could eat your way through life without bread.

But I was about to learn. I decided to take on this interesting project, and because I believe in living what I write, for me, that meant going gluten-free, totally and completely. Why? Because *you* have to go gluten-free, and I needed to feel your pain, work through your problems, and help you figure out what to order, what to buy, what to *eat*. As a food writer and avid home cook, food is very important to me, and I think it's probably very important to you, too. You want to know what to eat just as I do. So I decided to find the answers.

Over the next few months, I lived *your* life, playing the part of the gluten-intolerant hungry person in restaurants, at the grocery store, at the drive-through, even when eating with friends who cooked for me and didn't know that I couldn't (or wouldn't) eat gluten. I found out exactly what I could and couldn't eat, how to order off a menu without risking a gluten exposure, how to read a food label, how to get gluten out of my kitchen, and how to cook delicious meals without wheat, barley, or rye.

This book is the result of that experiment. You want to know what to eat, and we're here to tell you—that's my co-author, Tricia Thompson, M.S., R.D., a wonderful gluten-savvy nutritionist who has been eating gluten-free for 20 years, and me, Eve Adamson, your newly gluten-free food writer. Beyond this first chapter, we won't go much into why you can't eat gluten. Your doctor probably has told you all about that, or you've already read all the scientific details in other books or articles about gluten (for references to some of these and other great gluten-free resources, see Appendix B). Instead, we want to focus on the *food*, so you can start feeling a lot better and still look forward to dinner.

My Gluten-Free Adventure

On my first gluten-free day, I woke up, stretched, and wandered into the kitchen. I started a pot of coffee. My stomach grumbled, and I looked around. What the heck was I supposed to eat now?

Toast and jam would be nice. Or maybe some cereal. Wait a minute. Those won't do. They all have gluten—even that box of rice cereal in my pantry has wheat flour toward the end of the ingredients list and is flavored with malt syrup, which is made from barley. In other words: gluten.

Maybe I can have something a little heartier, like a breakfast burrito with some of that veggie sausage I have in the freezer. I surveyed the package: "This product contains wheat." What about the regular sausage? "Dextrose" and "flavoring" ... now, do those have gluten or not? I wasn't sure. (See Chapter 6 to find out.) Besides, I only had flour tortillas, and those won't do, either. I could run out for doughnuts? Croissant? Bagels? Rats! Gluten, gluten, gluten.

But wait a minute, I thought to myself. We're talking about bread, here. And pasta. And pizza. And chocolate chip cookies, for goodness sake! We're talking about a baguette with butter, birthday cake, and the bread basket at the restaurant. We're talking about croutons and macaroni and cheese and, and, and ...

After I finished my little gluten-deprivation tantrum (if you're already eating gluten-free, you know exactly what I mean), I decided to have some scrambled eggs to tide me over and then head to the grocery store. Surely the world is full of food without gluten. I just didn't have very much of it in my house! (In Chapter 2 you learn how to shop for gluten-free food.)

That's when I realized that eating gluten-free wasn't going to be easy and certainly not convenient. At least, not the way I was set up. I needed a book like this one ... a book that would tell me exactly what I could eat, until I got the hang of it, as I lived my life among people who ate gluten all the time, including my two sons and my "significant other," who weren't about to stop eating sandwiches and breakfast cereal just because I was writing a book.

In the meantime, I needed a little motivation. What's so bad about gluten, anyway? Isn't bread the "staff of life"? I wanted some good reasons to stop eating gluten because seriously ... can a little bread really be all that bad?

Why We Don't Tolerate Gluten

If you know, or even suspect, that your body has a problem with *gluten*, you may feel confused. You don't like feeling sick all the time, but you don't really understand why you can't eat something as basic as bread or pasta or crackers. Maybe you grew up thinking that soda crackers were the answer to an upset stomach or toast was the only thing you could eat when you were feeling sick. If you don't tolerate gluten, however, these are the worst possible foods for you to eat.

def•i•ni•tion ——————————————————————————

> **Gluten** is a protein found in wheat that gives dough its sticky, elastic quality. Some people have an autoimmune reaction to gluten and similar proteins in barley and rye. The word "gluten" has been used as an umbrella term to describe the proteins in wheat, barley, and rye that are harmful to people with celiac disease. While you may see references to corn gluten and rice gluten, these grains do not contain protein harmful to persons with celiac disease and are fine for you to eat.

Here's what happens: for some people, the proteins (generally called "gluten") in wheat, rye, and barley act like a poison in the small intestine. To protect itself, the body rebels, generating an autoimmune response against the gluten. In the process of this inner war, tiny nutrient-absorbing hairs in the small intestine called *villi* get eroded and eventually flattened.

When your villi are damaged, your body can't absorb the nutrients you need. Different people react to this malabsorption in different ways with different symptoms—and sometimes with no symptoms at all, even as internal damage rages on.

All that trouble can result from a slice of pizza and a mug of beer? Absolutely. According to the National Institutes of Health (NIH), up to one percent of Americans have *celiac disease*. That's about three million people, many undiagnosed or misdiagnosed with other problems like irritable bowel syndrome, diverticulitis, or chronic fatigue syndrome. Maybe you are one of them.

def•i•ni•tion ——————————————————————————

> **Villi** are microscopic little fingers of tissue on your intestinal wall covered with even smaller little protrusions called microvilli. Villi greatly increase your intestine's surface area so you can absorb digested nutrients more efficiently.
>
> **Celiac disease** is a genetic, autoimmune disease in which the body reacts to the proteins in wheat, rye, and barley (commonly called gluten) by damaging the intestinal *villi*, tiny hair-like protrusions in the small intestine that help absorb nutrients, resulting in problems absorbing nutrients. Celiac disease sometimes is called *celiac sprue, nontropical sprue,* or *gluten-sensitive enteropathy.*

Could You Be Gluten-Intolerant?

Everybody has an achy gut once in a while, but some people suffer chronic gastrointestinal problems or other generalized, vague-seeming symptoms of ill health. Some children stop growing, get very thin, and have mysterious health problems. If this sounds like you, your child, or someone in your family, you may be dealing with celiac disease, *gluten intolerance*, or *gluten sensitivity*.

def•i•ni•tion

Gluten intolerance and **gluten sensitivity** are non-specific terms that generally refer to an intolerance or sensitivity to gluten in wheat, barley, and rye, either because of celiac disease or for some other reason. Celiac disease and gluten intolerance are not allergies.

A **wheat allergy** is an allergic reaction specifically to wheat, rather than an autoimmune response to gluten. It is an acute condition that comes on within about two hours after eating wheat and is most common in children. People with wheat allergies can't eat wheat but can eat barley and rye.

If you have celiac disease and/or a gluten intolerance or sensitivity, you could have a wide variety of symptoms or no symptoms at all. Doctors used to think the main symptoms of celiac disease were gastrointestinal, and many people do have these kinds of symptoms when they eat gluten:

- Diarrhea
- Constipation
- Vomiting
- Nausea
- Bloating
- Gas
- Abdominal pain
- Unexplained weight loss

As scientists continue to study celiac disease, they are discovering the disease causes other symptoms and conditions that are not gastrointestinal in nature. One form of celiac disease, called *dermatitis herpetiformis*, manifests itself as a severe itchy rash. Other nongastrointestinal symptoms of celiac disease include:

◆ Migraines

◆ Numbness in the extremities

◆ Joint pain

◆ Fatigue

◆ Anxiety

◆ Depression

Infants and children with celiac disease also frequently experience:

◆ Small size

◆ Slow growth

◆ Failure to thrive

◆ Tooth enamel defects

◆ Developmental delays

◆ Delayed puberty

But treating your celiac disease means more to your health than just alleviating your uncomfortable symptoms—switching to a gluten-free diet actually could save your life. When you have celiac disease and your intestinal villi get flattened and destroyed, you can't absorb the nutrients you need to be healthy, and that can result in some really serious complications. If you have celiac disease and continue to eat gluten, you could develop any of the following complications, just to name a few:

◆ Iron-deficiency anemia

◆ Osteoporosis

◆ Infertility

◆ Miscarriage

◆ Intestinal lymphoma

◆ Adenocarcinoma

What does this mean for you? It means that if you think you might have celiac disease, you should get tested. Beyond the symptoms, other serious conditions have been associated with celiac disease, like thyroiditis, epilepsy, tuberculosis, and an increased chance of death from all causes at double the rate of the normal population. This is serious business, and if you have celiac disease, you want to know so you and your doctor can keep an eye on your health in the best possible way. If you don't have celiac disease, you may still decide to follow a gluten-free diet because it makes you feel better … but don't you want to know for sure?

Read the Label

If you have a family member with celiac disease or another autoimmune disease like type 1 diabetes, rheumatoid arthritis, thyroid disease, systemic lupus erythematosus, or Sjogren's syndrome, you may be at an increased risk for celiac disease. Ask your doctor if you should be tested.

Getting Tested for Celiac Disease

If you've picked up this book, you might already know for sure that you have celiac disease. Or maybe you don't know yet, but you are starting to wonder. You've heard about gluten and the problems it can cause. You've heard about the familiar symptoms. But you aren't too crazy about the idea of giving up wheat, so you are thinking: "Should I be tested?"

First of all, you have to be eating gluten before you get the celiac disease test—a major reason why many people who are already eating gluten-free don't want to get tested. You couldn't pay them to start eating gluten again.

But for those still eating gluten, getting tested for celiac disease is a three-step process. You have to "pass" all three steps before you can be officially diagnosed with celiac disease:

◆ Step one: you get a blood test (ask for the IgA antihuman tissue transglutaminase (IgA TTG) and IgA endomysial antibody immunofluorescence (IgA EMA) tests—that's a mouthful, but these are the tests currently recommended by the NIH as the most accurate.

◆ Step two: if your blood test shows you have antibodies for gluten, you will need a biopsy of your small intestine—a slightly unpleasant but minor outpatient procedure. Unfortunately, your doctor can't just look down there with some handy instrument. He actually has to snip out a piece from several different areas and take a good hard look at your intestinal villi so he can determine if they have been damaged, eroded, or utterly flattened. If they have, then you probably do have celiac disease, but the doctor still can't officially diagnose you until you complete step three. (If your doctor suspects you have dermatitis herpetiformis, the skin form of celiac disease, he will biopsy your skin rather than small intestine.)

◆ Step three: you stop eating gluten and feel better. Once that happens, your doctor can make an official diagnosis: you have celiac disease.

What your doctor recommends will depend on how all these tests come out. If you do have celiac disease, in a way, you are lucky. You don't need any drugs. You don't need any surgery. All you need is to follow a gluten-free diet for the rest of your life. You may not feel so lucky when you are craving a doughnut, but eating gluten-free is a lot easier and safer than many other treatments for other diseases.

But if your test results are negative or inconclusive (for example, a positive blood test but a negative biopsy), things can get a little more confusing. Your doctor may or may not say you are gluten-sensitive or gluten-intolerant and may or may not recommend a gluten-free diet. It all depends on the situation, so your doctor is the best one to advise you.

Fearless Eater

Before I wrote a word of this book, I made an appointment with my doctor and asked for a celiac test. The problem was that like many doctors, mine didn't know a lot about celiac disease. He had to look it up, and despite his good intentions, he ended up recommending the anti-gliadin antibody (AGA) test, a test no longer considered the best or most accurate test for celiac disease. Now I know what to ask for (the IgA TTG and IgA EMA tests). If you are given the wrong test and your doctor says you don't have celiac disease, but you are still feeling ill, then go back to the doctor and ask for the correct test.

Why You Shouldn't Diagnose Yourself

All the testing, doctor visits, and expense sounds pretty daunting, even if you've just about had it with the stomachaches and other problems you've been suffering. Right about now, you might be thinking, "Heck, it sounds like I have celiac disease. I'll just say I have it and start practicing a gluten-free diet right now."

But wait! Step away from the gluten-free bread!

Diagnosing yourself with celiac disease is a dangerous game. Celiac disease is very serious and can compromise your health in permanent ways, and it's true—a gluten-free diet is the one and only therapy and an effective therapy. But if you don't get tested and just "decide" you have celiac disease, you may not be as strict about your gluten-free diet. You may decide a little gluten here and there can't hurt when you are really craving a cookie or a sandwich. But for someone with celiac disease, this lapse can be very dangerous.

Or maybe you have some other serious condition that just seems to you to resemble celiac disease. If you feel something is wrong or if you are in poor health, it is very important *not* to diagnose yourself with celiac disease. If you put yourself on a gluten-free diet and feel a little bit better but still unwell, you could be ignoring something serious like lymphoma or intestinal cancer. Your self-diagnosis could prevent you from pursuing an actual diagnosis and keep you from seeking the treatment that could make you well again.

Some people argue that even without a diagnosis of celiac disease, if a gluten-free diet makes you feel better, then it won't hurt to follow it. If you don't test positive for celiac disease, only you and your doctor can decide together whether a gluten-free diet is appropriate for your individual situation. However, get tested first, just to be sure, and if you still feel sick, keep seeking an answer. In other words, please leave the diagnosis up to the experts.

Good for You

According to the NIH, there are no adverse nutritional outcomes associated with following a carefully planned gluten-free diet if you don't have celiac disease. However, keep in mind that celiac tests won't be accurate if you take them while following a gluten-free diet, so get tested before you stop eating gluten.

Gluten Intolerance: Not Celiac, Not Normal

All your tests came back negative, and your doctor says you don't (or probably don't) have celiac disease. So what's with the diarrhea, the bloating, the stomachaches, or the fatigue, the headaches, and the joint pain?

Some people have all the symptoms of celiac disease, but tests don't reveal anything wrong. If that sounds like you, then you might have a different problem unrelated to celiac disease. Or if going without gluten really does make you feel better, you and your doctor might decide that you are gluten-intolerant or gluten-sensitive, even without a diagnosis of celiac disease. Now what does that mean for you?

It means no more gluten, of course! Eating gluten and feeling bad without celiac disease may not be as life-threatening as eating gluten when you have celiac disease, but life threatening or not, why go through your life feeling bad?

This is really a matter of common sense. If something makes you feel bad, don't do it, whether or not you can put a name on the problem. If eliminating something from your diet makes you feel great, then do it, even if you don't have a diagnosis to 'justify' it. Listen to your body, and follow its lead. Even if your doctor says you don't have celiac disease, if your body says "Don't eat gluten!" then don't eat gluten. 'Nuff said.

The Verdict: No More Gluten

So that's the verdict: celiac disease or gluten intolerance or whatever the problem, gluten isn't for you. Now what are you supposed to do?

We know—you're hungry! That first gluten-free journey into the kitchen can be pretty daunting. Once upon a time, you might have whipped up a pot of pasta or a warmed up a frozen dinner or gone out for burritos and beer. But all that's off the list, now. What do you eat? What do you buy? What do you *order?* Is life worth living?

Have we got a surprise in store for you! There *is* delicious food beyond gluten. In fact, the gluten-free diet can be not only scrumptious but also interesting, fun to prepare, and a nutritional powerhouse, as well. You are going to feel *great*, and we dedicate the rest of this book to helping you embrace your new, gluten-free way of eating: how to cook, how to order, what to buy, and how to eat so you feel better than you've felt in a long time. Your gluten-free life is waiting. Are you ready?

The Least You Need to Know

◆ Gluten is a protein found in wheat but is often used as an umbrella term to describe proteins found in wheat, barley, and rye that people with celiac disease should not consume.

◆ Some people can't eat gluten because of a genetic condition called celiac disease. Gluten damages their small intestine so it can't absorb the nutrients it needs.

◆ To test for celiac disease, you must be eating gluten. If a blood test and an intestinal biopsy show you have celiac disease, your doctor will prescribe a gluten-free diet for the rest of your life.

◆ Some people aren't diagnosed with celiac disease but still have negative reactions to gluten. These people may be called gluten-intolerant or gluten-sensitive and may choose to follow a gluten-free diet.

◆ If you decide to give up gluten for any reason, this book will help you with all the practical aspects.

What's Got Gluten?

In This Chapter

- ◆ Foods not to eat
- ◆ Ways to spot gluten when the label doesn't make it obvious
- ◆ Check vitamins and pain relievers for gluten

So let's get right down to it. You're hungry, and you want to eat something, but you want something that doesn't contain gluten. And most of the stuff you have in your kitchen probably *does* contain gluten! So this chapter gets you started clearing out the old so you can bring in the new.

At first, it might seem like everything you want to eat contains gluten. That's how I felt ... no sandwiches (until I discovered gluten-free bread). No cookies (until I discovered gluten-free cookies). No burritos (until I discovered gluten-free tortillas). You see where I'm going with this ... you will learn there is much to eat! But first, we want to be sure you don't eat things that will make you sick. We want you to be able to walk into your kitchen and feel comfortable that any food you choose to eat (or order in a restaurant or enjoy at a friend's house) won't contain gluten. Consider this chapter your quick-and-easy rundown of the foods you must learn to live without to restore your health and live gluten-free.

Bread and Baked Goods

The first thing most people think about having to avoid when they learn they can't have gluten (or wheat) are the baked goods: bread, hamburger and hotdog buns, pizza crust, doughnuts, cookies, birthday cake … you know the food category we mean.

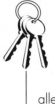

Good for You

As of January 1, 2006, life got a lot easier for people with celiac disease and others who can't eat wheat or gluten. The Food Allergen Labeling and Consumer Protection Act (which goes by the catchy acronym FALCPA) took effect on that date, and now, all foods regulated by the FDA *must* clearly list the presence of common allergens (milk, eggs, fish, crustacean shellfish, peanuts, tree nuts, soy, and yes, wheat) on the label in plain language anyone can understand.

It's true—this is the big, important category, the category that includes the foods you are probably most likely to crave, to miss, and to encounter everywhere you go. Most likely you are used to eating bread and baked goods all the time—most people are. But now you have to be more careful. You can't eat these things *if* they are made from wheat, rye, barley, or oats. (Unless the oats are gluten-free, but most aren't. We get more into that in Chapter 5, as well as in the next section about cereal.)

The good news is, you can buy or make most baked goods without gluten and many manufacturers committed to producing safe, gluten-free products make baked goods for your enjoyment. However, the lists in the next few sections include many of the specific baked goods you now need to avoid. This list isn't all-inclusive, but we want you to realize how many breads and baked goods contain gluten, so you can make smart choices the next time *you* want a sandwich or some pasta.

Bye-Bye, Bread (Except the Gluten-Free Kind!)

Staff of life, the soul of a sandwich, toast … whatever you want to call it or however you want to prepare it, bread is off-limits unless it's gluten-free. Gluten-free bread has come a long way, and while it doesn't taste like wheat bread, many people enjoy it.

But unless you know it is gluten-free, don't eat anything with the word "bread" in the name. The following list includes examples of the types of bread you should avoid. Bread goes by many names, so you must not eat any of the following or any foods made with the following (like bread stuffing, bread pudding, soup in a bread bowl, French toast, etc.):

◆ Bagels.

◆ Baguette.

◆ Breadsticks.

◆ Challa.

◆ Cornbread (the cornmeal part is okay but most cornbread also contains wheat flour).

◆ Croissants.

◆ Croutons (just order the Caesar salad without them).

◆ Dinner rolls.

◆ Dumplings.

◆ English Muffins.

◆ Flour tortillas, including whole wheat tortillas and flavored "wraps." (Corn tortillas and tortillas made by gluten-free manufacturers out of teff flour and rice flour are just fine.)

◆ Matzo.

◆ Multi-grain, mixed-grain, seven-grain, sprouted-grain, or any other "grain" bread (unless it is specifically gluten-free).

◆ Oatmeal bread.

◆ Pancakes, waffles, and French toast.

◆ Pita bread/pockets.

◆ Quick breads (like banana bread, zucchini bread, etc.).

◆ Rye bread (including marble rye).

◆ Rye crisps, cracker bread.

◆ Scones.

◆ Sourdough bread.

- ◆ Wheat bread.

- ◆ White bread.

- ◆ Whole wheat bread.

- ◆ Anything coated in "breading," like fried chicken, breadcrumb-coated fish, breaded cheese sticks, breaded hot wings, and batter-dipped anything (this includes almost every kind of appetizer and food they serve in "bar and grill" type restaurants, although an increasing number of restaurants now offer gluten-free options). Some places even batter-dip their french fries, so be sure to ask.

Fearless Eater

I went into my favorite bar-and-grill the other night and tried to figure out what I could eat and drink. My usual beer was off the list, so I ordered a gin martini instead. When the waitress came over to our table, I asked her if she had anything gluten-free. "That's wheat, right?" she asked, a little unsure of herself. "I don't think we have much." She was right—almost everything on the menu was dipped in batter and deep-fried, including the french fries. The only food on the menu that didn't contain some obvious source of gluten was the nachos—those had natural cheese, so that sounded good to me (but watch out for nachos with cheese *sauce*—ask the server if you can see the package label to look for wheat). I also ordered a side salad, hold the croutons, with oil and vinegar. I could have ordered a burger without the bun.

So Long, Cereal and Gluten-Containing Grains

Whether you can't face the day without your Frosted Flakes, you love beef-and-barley soup or tabbouleh salad for lunch, or you think a bowl of Raisin Bran makes a nifty nighttime snack, it's time to change your relationship to cereal.

You can buy gluten-free breakfast cereal made from corn, rice, or other gluten-free grains, but most mainstream cereals made from gluten-free grains, like crisp rice or flaked corn cereals, *do* contain gluten, either in the form of wheat flour or starch or, more commonly, in the form of malt syrup for flavoring (malt is made from barley, which contains gluten). As for the more savory grains, some will be just fine, but you must avoid several to stay gluten-free.

Read the Label _____

What about oatmeal? The more you read about gluten, the more you are likely to see references to the "oat argument." What's the issue? Well, most oats and oat products, including oatmeal and oat flour, are contaminated with gluten somewhere along the line from being grown in the field to being packaged. Even gluten-free oats can cause an immune reaction in a small minority of people with celiac disease. However, the FDA is proposing to allow gluten-free claims on oats that test less than 20 parts per million (of gluten). Some people with celiac disease eat small amounts of uncontaminated oats without any problems. However, until the term "gluten-free" is regulated and unless you get one of the few oatmeals out there guaranteed to be gluten-free (check out www.glutenfreeoats.com and www.pure-oats.com), that oatmeal on the grocery store shelf probably isn't gluten-free. For more about oatmeal, see Chapter 5.

That means no more:

◆ Cold cereal made from wheat, barley, rye, or most oats, or containing wheat flour, wheat starch, or anything containing the word "malt."

◆ Hot cereal, including farina (wheat) or cream of wheat, oatmeal (unless gluten-free), and malt-o-meal. Hot cereal made from rice or cornmeal (or any gluten-free grain) is fine as long as it doesn't contain any wheat, barley, rye, or malt flavoring.

◆ Wheat anything, including: wheat bran, wheat germ, wheat berries, wheat fiber, wheat starch, or wheat germ oil.

◆ Oat anything (unless gluten-free), including oat bran, oat fiber, oat flour, and oat starch.

◆ Pasta made from wheat, including semolina and durum wheat. That includes most mainstream varieties of spaghetti, linguine, fettuccine, penne, elbow macaroni, macaroni and cheese, ravioli, egg noodles, and pasta salad. (Pasta made from rice, corn, quinoa, or other gluten-free grains is fine.)

◆ Some Chinese and Japanese noodles, such as instant ramen noodles and any dishes containing lo mein, chow mein, and udon noodles. These are all made from wheat. Soba noodles are made from buckwheat, which would be okay except some of them also contain wheat flour, so look for the kind made from 100 percent buckwheat. The Chinese or Japanese noodles you _can_ eat include bean thread or cellophane noodles (made from mung bean starch) and rice noodles made with 100% rice flour. Also avoid egg rolls, wontons, and any other wrapped preparation unless you know it contains only rice paper or seaweed wrap, such as in sushi rolls.

- Couscous, a tiny pasta that looks like grain, commonly served with Middle Eastern cuisine.

- Orzo, a pasta that looks like rice (but isn't!)

- Dumplings. Ditch 'em—chicken soup is just as nice with rice.

- Gnocchi. Even though gnocchi is made with potatoes, it also uses flour to keep these little dumplings together.

- Barley. If your vegetable beef soup has those little barley grains floating in it, don't eat it.

- Bulgur. Most often found in Middle-Eastern dishes like tabbouleh salad, bulgur is a processed form of wheat that cooks quickly.

- Rye. Rye is most often found in rye bread and rye crisps. It has gluten, so eat the pastrami (gluten-free only, please) without it.

- Durum (sometimes called emmer), a kind of wheat often used in pasta. Sometimes it's called "durum wheat."

- Semolina, a coarsely ground durum wheat often used in pasta.

- Less common forms of wheat or wheat hybrids. You don't see these too often unless you hang out in the health food store, but avoid anything containing emmer (the same as durum), kamut, mir, einkorn, triticale, and spelt (sometimes called faro or dinkle).

Good for You

Buckwheat has the word "wheat" in it, but buckwheat isn't actually a type of wheat. Buckwheat groats and kasha (roasted buckwheat groats) are just fine for people following a gluten-free diet.

Good-Bye, My Sweets

We know, we know, sometimes you just have to have something *sweet*. That's fine, as long as it doesn't have gluten. Avoid all sweets made with wheat flour and/or sweetened with malt. For more on packaged food containing gluten, see Chapter 8. Meanwhile, avoid the following:

- Cake, including coffee cake and snack cake. (You can buy gluten-free cake mixes that taste delicious.)

◆ Cookies, homemade or store-bought, unless they say gluten-free (some of the packaged gluten-free cookies are pretty tasty).

◆ Brownies. If you just have to have chocolate, make fudge or flourless chocolate cake. Or purchase a gluten-free brownie mix.

◆ Doughnuts. Seriously, deep-fried gluten? Pass.

◆ Candy containing cookies, wafers, or cake. If the candy crunches or crumbles, suspect gluten. Demand purity in your candy!

◆ Any candy, cookies, or other sweets flavored with malt, including malted milk balls, malted milk shakes, and malted milk. Look for "malt" on the ingredients label for packaged baked goods and candy.

◆ Some ice cream, frozen yogurt, and flavored yogurt.

◆ Malts and malted milk.

Fearless Eater

The more I shop at the grocery store for gluten-free foods, the more I realize that many delicious foods are gluten-free just because they happen to be gluten-free, not because they are specifically manufactured to be that way. Fruits and vegetables, fresh chicken and fish and beef tenderloin, salad greens with olive oil and lemon juice, cheese, even snack foods like rice cakes (check the label to make sure they are gluten-free) and corn tortillas, almonds and walnuts, dried fruit, and bittersweet chocolate, have always been gluten-free. You still have to read the labels of any processed foods, and you will probably really appreciate foods that are manufactured to be gluten-free (like gluten-free pancake mix or cookies, for example), but don't forget about all the wonderful foods available that never had gluten and never will.

Baking Supplies

Those of us following a gluten-free diet learn to rely on products like gluten-free baking mix because baking can be tricky without wheat. (For "Secrets of a Gluten-Free Chef," see Chapter 12. For great sources of gluten-free baking mixes, see Chapter 9.) Meanwhile, avoid using any of the following in your gluten-free baking:

◆ Any flour made with wheat. If the label says "flour," that means wheat flour. Also avoid all-purpose flour, wheat flour, whole wheat flour, white flour, bread flour, cake flour, graham flour, and pastry flour.

◆ Matzo meal (made from wheat).

◆ Rye flour (rye also contains gluten).

◆ Oat flour, because it's usually contaminated with wheat.

◆ Wheat germ, wheat bran, or oat bran.

◆ Modified food starch, if it's made from wheat. It's often made from corn, however. According to recent FDA regulation, if modified food starch is listed on an FDA-regulated product and is made from wheat, it will say so on the label.

◆ Malt. It makes a nice flavoring, but it's usually made from barley, which contains gluten. Corn-malt is fine, but be sure you know what kind of malt you're consuming. If it just says "malt," avoid it.

No, Not Beer!

Most beer is made from malted barley, so it's full of gluten. This shocks and horrifies many of those new to the gluten-free diet, but we have great news—a few companies make gluten-free beer, and this small but growing category is now practically mainstream with the recent introduction of Redbridge, a sorghum-brewed beer from Anheuser-Busch. See Chapter 10 for more about gluten-free beers, and the results of my personal taste tests. You can also drink wine or any pure distilled liquor if you choose, even if it's made from grain, because the distilling process removes all the gluten. Some purists advise against liquor distilled from wheat, rye, or barley, but the fact is that no pure distilled liquor contains gluten. For more information about safe beer and other alcohol, see Chapter 10.

Processed Foods

If you cook everything from scratch, it isn't that hard to avoid gluten, but in this modern world, that can be tough. Processed food is everywhere, and it's fast and easy. But it also tends to be full of gluten.

However, you can avoid gluten if you know what to look for. The first thing to do is become an expert at reading food labels. For more about how to do this, see Chapters 4 and 5, and Chapter 8 on packaged food. In the meantime, every time you eat any packaged, processed food, you *must read the ingredient list*. It's the golden rule of gluten-free eating.

Fortunately, because of the recent law, all FDA-regulated products must list all common allergens in plain language, and that makes it a lot easier to spot sources of gluten. If any ingredient contains wheat, the ingredients list has to tell you that. So when you are reading an ingredients label on a processed food, you'll know to avoid any food that contains the following:

◆ Any item from any of the lists in this chapter.

◆ Anything that includes the word "wheat."

◆ Anything that includes the word "rye."

◆ Anything that includes the word "barley."

◆ Anything that includes the word "malt" or "malted," unless it specifically says the malt comes from corn. Anything that includes the word "oats" unless the oats are specially produced to be gluten free.

For more information about food ingredients, see Chapters 6, 7, and 8, which go into a lot more detail about processed foods and ingredients.

Good for You _____

Can you trust a product if it says it is "gluten-free"? Although the term "gluten-free" isn't currently regulated by the FDA, gluten-free manufacturers are usually caring, responsible, and ethical people who sincerely want to produce foods you can eat safely. Plus, gluten-free's unregulated status is about to change. A new ruling specifying an exact definition for the use of the term "gluten-free" will go into effect in 2008, so keep an eye on the website to follow the progress of this important regulation: www. fda.gov. For more information about gluten-free products and the use of this term, see Chapter 9.

Vegetarian Foods

We're not saying you *can't* be a gluten-free vegetarian, but it can be a challenge because the processed soy foods you might include as a staple in your diet (veggie burgers, veggie sausages, veggie chicken patties, veggie crumbles, etc.) mostly contain wheat gluten, which has a consistency similar to meat. Many veggie products also contain seitan, which is wheat gluten, or textured vegetable protein, which is usually made from wheat (the label will tell you what it is made from, according to FDA regulation). Of course, you can eat all the fruits, veggies, nuts, seeds, legumes, and plain unseasoned tofu you want. All of these are gluten-free, as long as they don't have any wheat, barley, rye, oat, or malt ingredients added to them.

Sorry, Snack Foods

Read the label for gluten ingredients. Many snack foods contain some kind of wheat, and many are flavored with malt. Of course, plenty of snack foods are just fine: popcorn, rice cakes, rice crackers, tortilla chips, nuts, seeds, dried fruit, and some "energy bars." (Read the label, though, just in case—some varieties of these products do contain gluten.) However, unless you know they are gluten-free, you'll definitely want to avoid any of the following:

- Snack cakes.
- Packaged cookies and brownies.
- Cereal bars and granola bars.
- Toaster pastries.
- Any candy containing cookies, wafers, cake, brownies, or malt flavoring.
- Pretzels.
- Crackers.
- Chips containing wheat, such as Sun Chips.
- Wheat nuts.
- Licorice.

Canned, Boxed, and Bottled Foods

Read the label for sources of gluten. Many sauces contain sources of gluten, especially Asian sauces. Condiments like ketchup, plain yellow mustard, and salsa are likely to be gluten-free, but read the label, just in case. Be particularly careful about the following:

- Bottled salad dressing.
- Soy sauce (many brands, but not all, contain wheat).
- Malt vinegar (regular distilled vinegar is okay).
- Teriyaki sauce, usually made with wheat.

- Gravy. Most are thickened with wheat flour.

- Soup. Most mainstream canned or jarred soups contain gluten, although if you read the labels, you can find soups without gluten, particularly some instant Asian soups with rice noodles. Or make your soup from scratch! (See Chapters 12 and 13.)

- Canned baked beans (some contain gluten but many do not).

- Instant rice mixes.

- Bouillon cubes.

- Instant cocoa or coffee mix (read the label—many are gluten-free).

- Fruit pie filling in a jar or can, includ-ing lemon curd (those thickened with tapioca or corn starch are fine—but make sure they aren't thickened with wheat flour or flavored with malt).

- Frozen vegetables in a sauce or with breading.

- Soy milk or other milk alternatives. Many are gluten-free, but read the label to be sure—some include wheat or barley (I don't know why, but they do).

 Read the Label

> Just because a product says it is wheat-free doesn't mean it is gluten-free. Wheat-free is a good start, sure, but don't forget to look for barley, rye, oat, or malt, too. These are all sources of gluten.

Farewell, Frozen Dinners!

Many frozen foods have long lists of additives and preservatives and they might be gluten-free, but read the label. If you see any ingredient containing wheat, barley, rye, malt, *or* oats (unless the product is processed to be gluten-free), pass. Most main-stream frozen dinners and even frozen vegetables in sauce contain gluten, so if you want to eat these foods, be vigilant. Watch out in particular for the following:

- Frozen dinners.

- Frozen vegetables in sauce.

- Frozen foods with breading.

- Frozen casseroles like lasagna, macaroni and cheese, or meatloaf.

Miss You, Meat! (At Least, the Processed Kind)

If it comes with a sauce, is injected with a basting solution, or is otherwise processed, read the label carefully for wheat ingredients or malt flavoring. In particular, read the labels for the following foods:

- Self-basting turkeys.

- Chicken (or any poultry) injected with any solution.

- Hot dogs, bologna, salami, pepperoni, cold cuts, and deli meat.

- Sandwich spreads, like tuna salad or ham salad.

- Sausage and bacon.

- Ham.

- Canned meat.

- Packaged meatloaf.

- Any meat with packaged gravy.

- Breaded fish/seafood or seafood packaged with sauce.

- Any meat or fish that comes with sauce, seasoning packets, or other flavoring.

Medications, Makeup, and Personal Products

Vitamins, herbal supplements, and over-the-counter medications sometimes might use gluten-containing ingredients as binders, fillers, and even dusting powders. Now, because of FALCPA, if a dietary supplement contains wheat, the manufacturer must list wheat on the label, and that can really ease the mind (and stomach) of someone with celiac disease.

For medications, however, it is important to call the manufacturer and ask if a product is gluten-free unless it says gluten-free on the label. Many of these products will have a phone number on them or at least a website where you can learn more.

For prescription medications, enlist the help of your pharmacist, who can either tell you if the product is gluten-free or call the manufacturer for you. Or you can always call the manufacturer yourself.

While cosmetics, lotions, and other personal care items can sometimes contain gluten, they shouldn't be harmful for someone with celiac disease unless there is a risk of actually ingesting the product, as with lipstick.

But if you want to be sure your new lip gloss doesn't contain gluten, call the manufacturer. For more information on gluten in nonfood items, check out Chapters 3 and 5.

The Least You Need to Know

- ◆ Many of the foods you have always eaten, from breads and flour tortillas to frozen dinners and teriyaki sauce, contain gluten. You'll need to eliminate these foods from your diet.

- ◆ Learn to read labels and recognize the obvious and not-so-obvious sources of gluten.

- ◆ Beware of food ingredients like malt flavoring, modified food starch made from wheat, and textured vegetable protein made from wheat.

- ◆ Some medications and cosmetics contain gluten, too. You or your pharmacist will have to call the manufacturer for assurance that a product is gluten-free.

Is Eating Gluten-Free *Really* Even Possible?

In This Chapter

◆ Get inspired to go gluten-free for good

◆ Prepare family and friends

◆ Check out the gluten-free products available out there

◆ Clear your house of the foods you can't eat

◆ Throw a gluten-free soiree to celebrate your new lifestyle (optional … but fun!)

After looking into the gluten-free diet, you might be feeling a little discouraged. What's left to eat? How will you live without your favorite comfort foods? Are you going to be a drag at parties? Are waiters going to be rolling their eyes at you?

Consider this your cheerleader chapter! You *can* go gluten-free, and you can even enjoy it. Go you! Rah rah rah!

Okay, that's not very helpful, we realize. That's why we devote this chapter to real-life strategies that *will* help you go gluten-free without feeling deprived, embarrassed, or a burden to the wait staff of the world. It just takes a little planning.

A New Way of Seeing

You can look at the world in two ways: full of delicious things you can't eat or full of delicious things you *can* eat. It's kind of a "glass half full" type of thing. You see, gluten-free manufacturers have worked hard to produce delicious products that can replace the gluten-full products you used to eat. But beyond that, many, many foods in the world are naturally gluten-free. They have never contained gluten, and you might have forgotten all about them because you've been too busy mourning the loss of your morning toast.

Let's think about this for a minute: sweet, juicy fruit. Tender, savory vegetables. Delicious rice pilaf made with basmati, jasmine, yellow rice, wild rice, brown rice … or better yet, risotto! Creamy, perfect food.

And what about meat? Imagine the mouthwatering aroma of a roasting chicken, a sizzling loin of beef, a perfectly prepared salmon filet drizzled with olive oil and dill, perhaps with a side of creamy garlic mashed potatoes and broccoli sizzled in oil with hot pepper flakes or cheese. You can eat Asian rice noodles with chili oil and sesame seeds or stir-fry. You can even have wine or a mixed drink if you prefer.

You can also drink milk, sample the finest French cheeses, eat ice cream with chocolate syrup or a banana split, dip your spoon into pudding, frozen yogurt, or a lovely mousse. You can have rice cakes with almond butter and cherry jam, tostadas with black bean chili, homemade chicken soup with rice, even nachos! Okay, now we're getting really hungry.

And we haven't even mentioned spaghetti, lasagna, and all the other delicious pasta dishes you can make with rice or quinoa pasta (or any other gluten-free pasta). You can also have warm, comforting rice cereal or cold crispy cereal made with sorghum, rice, or corn. And if you really miss your toast, start sampling the different gluten-free breads, or make your own. So you see, things aren't so bad. They might be a little different, but you can do this! You aren't going to starve—far from it. In fact, you're going to be feeling pretty satisfied, we promise. You just have to get started.

The First Ten Things to Do

You know those quick-start instructions you get whenever you buy a new piece of electronic equipment like a digital camera or a DVD player? Or TiVo? The ones that get you up and running before you have time to go through the whole instruction manual?

We love those, and we want you to feel completely comfortable from the beginning of your new gluten-free diet in just that way. So here is your quick-start instruction manual—the first 10 things you can do, or plan, *right now* to get you up and running on your gluten-free diet. Are you ready?

(1) Adjust Your Attitude

This first step is very important. You need to be ready to do this, so you don't get careless or tempted to cheat. This is about your health. If you aren't healthy, you can't be any good to others, and you won't be able to get the most out of your own potential. *Your health matters.*

So every time you get angry or tempted or otherwise want to throw in the gluten-free towel, we want you to have a phrase you can repeat, to reinspire you and remind you how important this is. You need something short and sweet, something to-the-point that speaks to you and that you can say to yourself. Your mantra might be any of the following:

- My health matters.
- I will take care of myself.
- Health feels good.
- I will stay in balance.
- Gluten hurts; gluten-free helps.
- Gluten-free helps me be a better [parent, wife/husband, friend, caretaker, world peace initiator, or whatever works for you].

And of course, what these all mean is that you won't eat gluten. You don't have to use one of these—you can make one up for yourself. The point is to have something to say when your attitude or will starts to slip. Repeat it often.

(2) Call a Family Meeting

You can take yourself in hand and dedicate yourself to the gluten-free life, but what about the rest of your family? If you have celiac disease, chances are, some of your immediate relatives have it, too, and should be tested. But those who don't have it may have a hard time understanding or getting on board with your new prescription.

As my kids like to say to me, "Why should *we* have to eat gluten-free just because you're writing that weird book?" Ah, youth. The fact is, they *love* the gluten-free chocolate chip pancakes I've been making, and they can't tell the gluten-free brown rice cereal from the malt-flavored stuff they were eating before. And as for dinner, they can eat their burgers on buns. I like mine atop a crispy corn tortilla.

But still, you're going to want to lay down some rules, so this calls for a family meeting. Get the crew together (even if "the crew" is just one other person) and sit them down. Explain what your diagnosis means for you and the family. Explain that even a little bit of gluten could make you sick and compromise your health and that you will need everyone's support to help you stay healthy and strong. Then, you can remind them that *they* can eat gluten, but they should never try to get *you* to eat it—ever again. And tell them that you will appreciate their understanding and support. This will help you feel like you aren't in this alone and that the people who love you will be there to help you along.

 Read the Label

One concern about going gluten-free when you live with others who aren't gluten-free is cross-contamination. Is your beloved getting toast crumbs all over your butter? Are your kids dipping their crackers in your strawberry jam? Same goes for peanut butter, mustard, mayonnaise, and anything else that gluten-eaters share with you. To guard against this, make it clear to everyone in the family that you must have separate gluten-free versions of these foods: butter or margarine, nut butters, jams and jellies, and all condiments. Or consider investing in squeeze-bottle versions.

(3) Trash the Bad Stuff

Step three is fun. Take a garbage bag, and head into the kitchen. Take a good look around. If everyone in the household is going gluten-free, then take everything with gluten and throw it into the trash. Or put it into a bag or box to give to a non-gluten-sensitive friend. Or donate unopened products to a local food pantry. Empty your kitchen of:

- ◆ Bread.

- ◆ Crackers.

- ◆ Flour tortillas.

- ◆ Baked goods of every kind.

- ◆ Cold breakfast cereal containing wheat, barley, rye, oats (unless gluten-free), or malt.

- ◆ Oatmeal (unless gluten-free variety).

- ◆ Wheat flour (including white flour and all-purpose flour).

- ◆ Packaged processed food with wheat, barley, rye, oats, or malt.

- ◆ Beer (unless gluten-free variety).

- ◆ Anything else with wheat, barley, rye, oats, or malt.

- ◆ Anything that contains pasta made from wheat (that includes semolina and those pretty vegetable-colored pastas).

Yes! We know! This is hard! It seems like a waste of money, too. But just remember, as far as *your* body is concerned, you are throwing out poison. Poison is bad. Get rid of it. Starting now, you'll only spend your money on food that will nourish you.

If people in your household are still eating gluten, throw away all the things you know they don't eat, that are really yours (the whole-wheat tortillas? Or are you more the doughnut type?). Put all the other gluten-full stuff in one cabinet. You might even label it the "gluten cabinet." They can help themselves.

(4) Explore the Grocery Store

Agent GF (that's Gluten-Free), we have a reconnaissance mission for you. You are to travel to the grocery store and explore the lay of the gluten-free land. Report back at your convenience. This message will not self-destruct.

The first time you go to the grocery store, you don't have to buy a thing. This really is a reconnaissance mission, and it might take some time, so give yourself a couple of hours. (Or less if you really can't stand the grocery store—it's one of my favorite places so I go there a lot just to hang out. Is that weird? Wait, don't answer that.)

Go through the aisles and note all the good things you can eat, and notice all the things you might have gotten before but can't eat anymore. Pick up packages. Read labels. The first time you do it, this will be a real education. You won't believe how interesting a food label is when it really matters to your health! (For more information on reading food labels, check out Chapter 4.)

Look for the gluten-free section. Many stores put the gluten-free specialty products all together, for easy browsing. See what they have. You may never have noticed this section before! I was surprised to find how many gluten-free specialty products my regular old grocery store stocked: Brownie mix! Crackers! Frosted cereal! Macaroni and cheese in a box! *Cookies*! (I got very excited.)

And remember, plenty of foods are *naturally* gluten-free, so you will be able to find them all over the store. Are you getting inspired yet?

Good for You

If your regular grocery store doesn't have much in the way of gluten-free foods, check out the local health food store, food co-op, or one of the new big main- stream stores like Whole Foods and Wild Oats. Both of these stores have lots of delicious gluten-free foods, from muffins, biscuits, and scones to pizza crust, sand- wich bread, and dinner rolls. Look here to see what they have before you head out to the store:

- ◆ Whole Foods: www.wholefoodsmarket.com/products/bakery/gf_bakehouse.html
- ◆ Wild Oats: www.wildoats.com/u/department165

(5) Surf the 'Net for the Food You Can't Find

We hope you found your trip to the grocery store stimulating or at least a little bit inspiring. But maybe you didn't find some of the things you were hoping to find. Maybe you live in a small town, and your store doesn't have many gluten-free prod- ucts, and you're just dying for a sandwich or some quinoa spaghetti. Lucky for you, many gluten-free manufacturers sell their products online. To get you started brows- ing from the comfort of your own home, look here:

- ◆ The Gluten-Free Mall. You can find tons of great products here: www.gluten- freemall.com.

- ◆ Gluten-Free Food Vendor Directory. This site lists lots of different gluten-free product manufacturers, with links to their sites so you can buy direct: www. gfmall.com.

◆ Allergy Grocer. This fun site lets you search according to your allergy or the ingredient you don't want in your food. You can also search specifically for kid-friendly products, which is super helpful if your kids can't eat gluten: www.allergygrocer.com.

(6) Give Your Medicine Cabinet a Facelift

If you take vitamin/mineral supplements or other supplements like glucosamine for arthritis or probiotics for digestion or herbal supplements for whatever reason, you need to find out if they contain gluten. According to law, supplements that contain wheat must state this, so in most cases, you can find out by reading the label, unless the supplement was manufactured before 2006. But if that's the case, your supplements are probably expired. Check the date!

Medications don't have to follow that same rule, however. They may contain a wheat-based ingredient and don't have to say so. That goes for over-the-counter medicine (like an antihistamine) or for prescription medicine. You might see lists on the Internet or in books that give vitamin, supplement, and drug manufacturers who are gluten-free, but some of these may be outdated and companies can change their ingredients at any time.

So for this step, collect all the supplements and medications you ever take, and look on the packages for information about the product's ingredient and gluten content. If you don't see this information, look for the manufacturer's contact information. If you can't find it, search for the manufacturer or the product name on the Internet to find the contact information. Sometimes the website will tell you if the product is gluten-free, but sometimes you'll have to call and ask. Make a list of who you need to call.

(7) Flex Your Phone Finger

Once you've got your list of supplement/medication manufacturers' phone numbers, it's time to start calling. Don't put it off! You might as well get used to doing this, because sometimes it's necessary. Call them, one by one, and tell the person who answers the phone that you need to know if Product X or Medication Y contains wheat or barley. For more information on finding out about the gluten status of non-food items, see Chapter 5.

(8) Break the News to Your Friends

You've talked to your family. You've cleaned out your cabinets. But what are your friends going to think? When you go gluten-free, all the people in your life should know—at least, the ones who might cook for you or eat with you in the future. Invite your best buds out for coffee or tea (both, thankfully, entirely gluten-free, although read the label on any mixes or flavored varieties) and lay it out for them: you can't eat gluten any more, and although they might think it's strange, if they are your friends and want you to be healthy and feel good, they will understand and not make it harder for you. You'll want to make a couple of general points to your friends (but of course, your friends are *your* friends, so adjust this list as it's relevant for you). Explain to them that:

◆ You can't eat anything with wheat, rye, barley, or oats (unless gluten-free), and that includes all the products people generally think of as containing flour, including bread (your friends may gasp) and pasta (don't be surprised if someone faints).

◆ You won't be offended by other people eating gluten; you just can't have gluten in your own diet.

◆ When you all eat together, you can't share food with gluten, and you can't even eat food prepared in a pan that just cooked something with gluten. If somebody has a dinner party, tell her you will be more than happy to bring something for yourself so she won't have to prepare something different for you.

◆ Explain that you aren't being picky, you are only doing what you've been told is necessary for your health.

Many people are curious about what all this means. They may not know what kind of foods contain gluten or what gluten is. If they have more questions, refer them to this book, a great tool for people who love someone who is gluten-intolerant.

Fearless Eater

When you quit eating gluten, you may have to break it gently to your beer-drinking buddies. I wrote a book on craft beer last year, and my beer-snob friends, well ... they weren't very understanding, but when I got them interested in gluten-free beer tasting, they came around. Tell your buddies you can bring gluten-free beer to the next party for yourself. (For more information about gluten-free beer, see Chapter 10—I rated the main ones I could find, so you'll want to check it out if you love beer like I do!)

(9) Go Out to Eat: A Practice Run

Eating gluten-free in a restaurant can be a real adventure. Some restaurants are ready for you, and some aren't. When I first ate gluten-free in my favorite sushi restaurant, I asked if they had wheat-free soy sauce. The confused waitress told me that soy sauce doesn't contain wheat. I showed her the bottle, and pointed to the word "wheat"—the second ingredient. She pointed at the low-sodium soy sauce, and said happily, "You can have this, it's low-sodium!" Again, I pointed to the word "wheat." She just stared at me for a minute, then said, bleakly, "You mean, you can't eat bread?" She patted my shoulder, then walked away, which didn't help me with my quest for a salty condiment to enjoy with my salmon sashimi.

You won't know about the gluten-free status of your food in a restaurant until you ask. Sometimes, you might have to talk to the chef yourself, although most wait staff are accommodating. Sometimes, you might have to ask to see a package or bottle if you can't get the right information. Sometimes, you might not have very many options and you might get tired of eating salad with a broiled chicken breast. (But was it cooked on a pan that just cooked a breaded chicken breast? You'll have to ask.) Some wait staff will roll their eyes at you, but others are wonderfully accommodating. Go out to eat tonight, if you can, and start practicing. There's no time like the present.

For more information on eating in restaurants, including the gluten-free status of some of your favorite restaurant meals, see Chapter 15.

Fearless Eater

The first time I went into a restaurant after I went gluten-free, I told the waitress I had to be sure none of the food I was eating contained any wheat. She said, "Oh, do you have a gluten allergy?" Some people mistakenly call celiac disease or gluten intolerance a "gluten allergy." This is a misnomer—celiac disease is not an allergy. However, because it was a nice restaurant and I didn't feel the need to get into a long technical discussion geared toward waitress re-education, I just said "Yes." She smiled and was very accommodating, making sure nothing I ate had gluten and the rolls were on the opposite end of the table where I didn't have to smell them. (It didn't keep my boyfriend from eating them in front of me, of course.)

---

(10) Throw a Gluten-Free Gala!

All this preparation might seem like a lot to do, but you've adjusted your attitude, remember (see Step 1), so you're enjoying it, right? Even if you feel a little bit put-upon by all this extra work (or especially if you do), you might consider throwing a gluten-free party. This is your chance to practice cooking some basic gluten-free appetizers, talk to friends about how things are going, and see how much fun it can be to party without the gluten. Big or small, 2 friends or 20 or 200 (whatever you're up for), a party can be a great opportunity to increase the good buzz about your new lifestyle.

Some suggested refreshments:

- Wine, champagne, mixed drinks, or freshly squeezed juice cocktails

- Dates stuffed with goat cheese and wrapped with strips of pancetta or thinly sliced bacon (read the label to make sure the pancetta and bacon are gluten-free)

- Corn tortillas baked with a little olive oil, garlic powder, and salt, broken or cut into wedges, and served with fresh salsa and homemade guacamole (mash avocadoes with a little salsa, lime juice, and freshly chopped cilantro)

- Deviled eggs (boil eggs, scoop out yolks, mix with a little mayonnaise and pickle relish, return to egg halves, sprinkle with paprika)

- A selection of gluten-free cookies and brownies from the store, either premade or from a mix that you make yourself, so you can sample them and choose your favorites

For more interesting and fun ideas for cooking gluten-free, see Chapter 12.

Now, don't you feel integrated into the gluten-free lifestyle? But wait ... we have so much more to share with you, so stay with us. We won't leave you to your own devices just yet.

The Least You Need to Know

- Giving up gluten is easier if you have a positive attitude about your new lifestyle.

- Get started by taking 10 easy steps to start you on the right path.

- Tell your family and friends about your new lifestyle and why it is important for you to be gluten-free, so you have a support system.

- Start learning where to find gluten-free foods, and get rid of the foods you can't eat so they won't tempt you.

◆ Get out there in the world and be gluten-free in public. Eating in restaurants is always an adventure and takes some practice. Eating at a friend's house might mean bringing your own dish.

◆ To practice all your new gluten-free strategies, throw a party. Serve all gluten-free foods. Your friends probably won't even notice.

Part 2

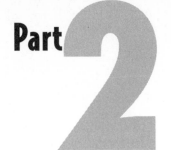

What to Eat and
What to Avoid

The grocery store can be a confusing place when you can't eat gluten. Never fear, Part 2 is here! This is the place to find out how to decipher that food label, where gluten could be hiding, and what manufacturers are legally required to reveal on the package label. You'll also get helpful lists of foods that you can probably eat safely, with explanations for each item, and foods you should probably avoid, also with explanations (because we often find exceptions whenever we try to put an item on a list).

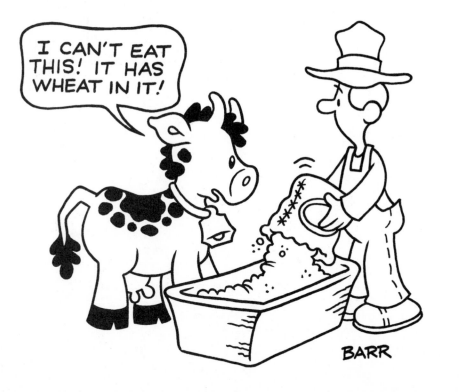

Chapter 4

How to Read a Food Label

In This Chapter

◆ Information food labels can and can't give

◆ The ins and outs of ingredients lists

◆ The laws about food allergens and food labels, and ways they help you (even if you don't have any food allergies)

◆ Finding sources of wheat, rye, and barley on a food label

It doesn't seem fair. Some people can pick out a food that looks good, and just, just … eat it. No problem! They won't pay for their cavalier attitude with nausea or getting stuck in the bathroom for an hour. Sure, they might put on a few extra pounds or get indigestion once in a while, but that seems a small price to pay for the luxury of eating anything they want without having to make a big production about reading the label or grilling the poor server, who may not even know what gluten is.

You, on the other hand, have to read the food label before you put anything in your mouth. You have to grill the server. You have to *know*. Sometimes that can be a drag. Believe us, we understand!

However, let's look at this in a whole different light. Maybe you're in the better position, because maybe, just maybe, unenlightened eating isn't such a great thing. And maybe reading a food label can be downright interesting!

I think it is. In fact, I've taken to doing it just for fun, even when I *know* a product is gluten-free.

If you are what you eat, don't you want to know what you are eating?

In fact, being an enlightened label reader makes you a more enlightened eater, so you'll be aware of not only what foods contain gluten, but also how much fat, calories, artificial ingredients, or healthy ingredients are in the foods you eat. If you ask us, everybody should become a label reader. How else can you intelligently avoid trans fats, for example, or high fructose corn syrup or artificial colors and preservatives, if you don't want to put those things into your body? How else will you know if a product is, for example, organic or fiber-rich, or has enough calcium to help you meet your daily requirement?

Okay, we know, this isn't a book about nutrition so we'll save our lectures about healthy eating for another book (and for Chapter 17, where we talk about maintaining a healthy weight on a gluten-free diet) and won't digress too much right now.

The point is that reading food labels is in everybody's best interest, and to do it well, you have to know a little bit about how food labels work and what they can and can't say. This chapter is here to help.

Besides, reading a label and finding out your favorite instant latte mix doesn't contain gluten will put you in a much better mood than reading all those depressing stories in the newspaper. Want some light reading over breakfast? Let's do it!

The Anatomy of a Food Label

Food labels accomplish several important things. They tell you how many calories are in a product. They tell you basic nutritional information, like how many grams of fat, carbohydrates, and protein a product has in it. They tell you what a serving size of that product is and how many servings the package contains. They also have to list all the ingredients in a product (according to certain guidelines), so you know exactly what you are eating.

If you are a food manufacturer and you make a product, it is regulated by the *Food and Drug Administration*, a.k.a the FDA (unless it's meat, poultry, or egg products in which case it's regulated by the United States Department of Agriculture or USDA). The FDA has rules about how food labels must be set up and what they can and can't say. For instance, the food label can't make claims that aren't true. Terms like "low-fat" or "organic" are strictly regulated—you can't put them on the label unless you follow all the rules associated with that term.

def•i•ni•tion

The Food and Drug Administration (FDA) is a part of the United States Department of Health and Human Services. Their primary purpose is to regulate food and drug products to protect human health. The FDA works hard to ensure that the foods we eat and the medicines we take are safe. To find out more about the FDA, check out their website at www.fda.gov.

Reading food labels used to be complicated for people who have to avoid gluten, but thanks to the Food Allergen Labeling and Consumer Protection Act (also known as FALCPA), things are much easier. The part of FALCPA relevant for people who can't eat gluten is just this: if a product contains wheat protein, the word "wheat" has to be included on the food label. Wheat can't hide anymore. And that's good news. (See the section about wheat later in this chapter.)

But reading a food label effectively takes a little more knowledge than just looking for the word "wheat" (although that's a big part of what you need to know). Food labels must contain an *ingredients list* that has to follow specific guidelines. Also, in the case of foods containing major allergens like wheat, a "CONTAINS" statement may be present below the ingredients list if the ingredients list doesn't make the presence of the allergen absolutely clear.

Good for You

Technically, a product can't say "gluten-free" if it isn't gluten-free. However, until recently, the term "gluten-free" didn't have any published rules dictating exactly what it meant, so manufacturers could put the term on a product without specific rules about its use. Now, however, the FDA is working on specific guidelines to regulate the term, which will make the words "gluten-free" on a package of food more meaningful. As this book went to press, the rules weren't officially in place yet, but by the time you read this, they may be in force. For the latest news, check out the FDA's website at www.fda.gov, and type "gluten-free" in the search field for the latest updates. Also check out Chapter 5 for more information about the term "gluten-free."

Ingredients Lists

Every packaged food product must have an ingredients list if it is made from two or more ingredients, so you know exactly what you are eating. Even products with just one ingredient have to contain an ingredients list if that ingredient is a common allergen, according to FALCPA. But the manufacturer can't just list the ingredients any way it wants—it can't put the healthiest ingredients first, just for the purpose of making the product look healthy. It can't put healthy ingredients in bigger text, either. We have rules, people!

One good thing to know is that the ingredients list must be in order of how prevalent each ingredient in the product is by weight. The product contains more of the first ingredient listed than any other ingredient. And contains the least of the last ingredient.

For example, I'm looking at a can of spaghetti sauce. This is what the ingredients list says:

> TOMATO PUREE (WATER, TOMATO PASTE), WATER, LESS THAN 2% OF: MUSHROOMS, HIGH FRUCTOSE CORN SYRUP, SALT, CORN SYRUP, SOYBEAN OIL, SUGAR, DEHYDRATED ONIONS, CARROT FIBER, CITRIC ACID, SPICES (INCLUDING SOY LECITHIN), NATURAL FLAVOR.

Fearless Eater

I have a lot of favorite foods, and many of them are now off-limits. However, sometimes things work out just fine. I was so pleased, recently, to read the label on my favorite Thai Kitchen Pad Thai mix:

Rice Noodles (Rice, Water), Sauce Packet (Sugar, Tomato, Natural flavor, Radish, Anchovy Extract, Water, Garlic, Salt, Paprika). Manufactured in a facility that uses peanuts.

And finally, much to my surprise, guess what it says, right there on the box under the ingredients statement? (Drum roll …) Yep, "GLUTEN-FREE." Wow, and I've been buying this since way before I knew what gluten even was.

This means that this particular can of spaghetti sauce contains more tomato puree than anything else, because that is listed first. It also contains water, but not as much water as tomato puree, because the water is listed second. Notice that "high fructose corn syrup" and "corn syrup" are listed separately. Lump them together and they might be higher up in the ingredients list, but because they are slightly different, they can be listed separately. This spaghetti sauce also contains natural flavor, but the amount of natural flavor is less than the amount of any other product because that ingredient is listed last.

Also, notice that after "SPICES" it says "(INCLUDING SOY LECITHIN)." The reason this one ingredient in spices is specified is because soy is a common allergen. FALCPA says that it therefore must be clearly labeled (see the next section for more information about allergen labeling). If those spices contained wheat, it would have to say that, too.

As for that natural flavor, it could possibly contain trace amounts of malted barley and, therefore, trace amounts of gluten. However, it probably doesn't. For more information about why it probably doesn't, and other considerations regarding hidden glutens in ingredients like natural flavors and what you probably do and probably don't have to worry about, see Chapter 5.

Let's look at another, more obvious gluten-relevant example. I have a can of chicken noodle soup in front of me, and this is what the ingredients list says (I won't list the whole thing because it's too long—just one more reason, as far as I'm concerned, to make your soup from scratch):

> INGREDIENTS: CHICKEN STOCK, COOKED ENRICHED EGG NOODLE PRODUCT (WHEAT FLOUR, EGG WHITE, EGG, NIACIN, FERROUS SULFATE, THIAMINE MONONITRATE, RIBOFLAVIN, FOLIC ACID), CARROTS, WATER, CONTAINS LESS THAN 2% OF THE FOLLOWING: COOKED CHICKEN MEAT, MODIFIED FOOD STARCH, CELERY, SALT …

Now you know the ingredient the soup contains the *most* of is chicken stock. The second most prevalent ingredient is cooked enriched egg noodle product. Notice that after this, in parenthesis, is a secondary list of ingredients for the egg noodle product. This list is also in order of amount. The noodle product has more wheat flour than anything else. And notice that they say "wheat flour" instead of "flour." Because of FALCPA, they can't just say "flour" on an ingredients label anymore because wheat is a common allergen. They have to say "wheat flour" so the wheat-allergic can recognize that the product contains wheat (and therefore, gluten**)**.

There are exceptions to this rule. If more than one ingredient in a food product contains wheat, wheat only has to be identified for one ingredient, not for all. Also, wheat may not be identified at all within the ingredients list if the manufacturer chooses instead to use a "CONTAINS" statement. Rest assured, however, that if wheat protein is in a food product regulated by the FDA, the word "wheat" will be included on the food label somewhere.

Because the soup clearly states in the ingredients label that it contains wheat and egg (two of the most common allergens), it doesn't include a "CONTAINS" statement after the ingredients list, but the manufacturer could have chosen to include one. Many do. (See the next section.)

And in case you're wondering about the "modified food starch," it's probably made from corn, and if it were made from wheat, it would have to say so … but see Chapter 5 for more information about that.

"CONTAINS" Statements

As we've already explained, FDA-regulated products have to list all their ingredients in an ingredients list. If they contain any of the eight major food allergens, they must also, by law, list the presence of those allergens very clearly, either in the ingredients list or in something called a "CONTAINS" statement. Many products use both. Flavorings, colorings, and spices can be listed collectively, but they also have to say if any of them contain wheat or other allergens, or the allergens must be listed in a "CONTAINS" statement.

You might see the "CONTAINS" statement listed after the ingredients list like this: ALLERGY INFORMATION or ALLERGEN INFORMATION. For instance, I have a bag of gluten-free baking and pancake mix right here on my desk. (I don't normally keep it here, in case you're wondering.) After the ingredients list, it says:

> ALLERGEN INFORMATION: CONTAINS TREE NUTS AND MILK.

That can of spaghetti sauce I was looking at in the last section has a "CONTAINS" statement instead. After the ingredients list, it says:

> CONTAINS: SOY

According to the law, the word "CONTAINS" must be located immediately following or next to the list of ingredients, and at least the first letter in the statement must be in caps, although many manufacturers put the whole statement in capital letters and in bold. Also, the law says the letter size cannot be any smaller than the ingredients list. In many cases, you'll find it is larger.

Read the Label

According to the FALCPA law, the eight major food allergens, which account for 90 percent of all food allergies, are milk, eggs, fish, crustacean shellfish, peanuts, tree nuts, wheat, and soy.

The purpose is to make things easier for people with allergies. Even though celiac disease and gluten intolerance aren't allergies, those of us with this condition benefit greatly because of the FALCPA law. The "CONTAINS" statements don't list other sources of gluten, like rye, barley, and malt. But because wheat is the main source of gluten in most processed foods, this information really helps those of us who eat gluten-free.

Manufactured in a Facility That Contains ...

When you spend your free time reading food labels, you begin to notice a lot. Not only are ingredients labels, nutritional content, "CONTAINS" statements, and the pretty pictures all interesting, but you might also notice that some products, including gluten-free products, have a statement about being manufactured in a facility that also manufactures various allergens like peanuts, milk, or wheat. Should this concern you?

Probably not ... but maybe (don't you hate answers like that?). Manufacturers put this statement on their products, not because they have to by law, but, most likely, for liability reasons. All manufacturers are supposed to follow standards of good manufacturing practice, which includes thoroughly cleaning equipment to prevent contamination from other food products. If the machine making your gluten-free bread also bakes regular bread (for example), the manufacturer is supposed to be darned sure no bread residue remains from one loaf to the next. The FDA also periodically tests food products for cross-contamination and inspects facilities for evidence of good manufacturing practices. However, you can imagine that it would be possible to get a little bit of cross-contamination. Would it be enough to make you sick? Maybe. Maybe not. And it's also quite possible that the equipment *is* thoroughly cleaned and no gluten residue remains at all.

If given a choice, people with celiac disease would probably choose a gluten-free product made in a dedicated gluten-free facility over one made in a facility that also processes products made from wheat. The simple fact is that whenever you eat a processed food, you always run a slight risk of contamination. Are you willing to take the risk? Only you can answer that question. Many people are. Many people aren't. Fortunately, a lot of food labels give you the information you need to make that decision yourself.

The Many Faces of Wheat

Before FALCPA, wheat could be contained in a food without the food necessarily specifically stating this. A food might list "flour" or "modified food starch," without saying the word "wheat." Also, different wheat species and hybrids could be listed under different names, like triticale, emmer, spelt, semolina, and kamut. But no more!

FALCPA requires any kind of wheat to be labeled as "wheat," and any food ingredients containing wheat to say so. Now a product has to say "wheat flour" or "made from wheat." Or it might put the wheat in parentheses, like "modified food starch (wheat)." The point is, if it has wheat, it has to say so. Just remember that it may not say so on the front of the label. *You have to look at the ingredients list and the "CONTAINS" statement.*

Rye Humor

Rye isn't the most common grain out there, but you will see it in some products. Fortunately, in most cases, rye is labeled as rye because many people like the taste and food manufacturers want people to know it's in there.

Some of the food products that contain rye are rye bread, rye crisp crackers, and some mixed-grain breads and cereals. Read the label, and you'll find out if any of those "mixed grains" contain rye (they probably also contain wheat and possibly barley). A few varieties of beer contain rye in addition to barley, making them full of gluten.

Fearless Eater

I love vintage cocktails. The more history to a cocktail, the more I want to try it. I once spent a whole evening in New Orleans (prehurricane) trying to find the Sazerac hotel so I could try their signature cocktail, the Sazerac. One of the main ingredients in the Sazerac cocktail, as well as many other vintage cocktails like some versions of the Manhattan, the Millionaire Cocktail, and the Preakness, is rye whiskey. Off limits for the gluten-intolerant? Imagine how happy I was to discover that even though rye whiskey (and other liquors) are made from gluten-containing grains, the distilling process banishes all the gluten. Bartender, I'll have another …. (For more information on the alcoholic beverages you can and can't drink, see Chapter 10.)

Barley and Malt: The Gluten Sneaks

Honestly, wheat really is your biggest concern when it comes to eating gluten-free just because it is in so many foods. However, another significant source of gluten in the standard American diet is barley, mostly in the form of *malt*.

Malt or malted barley is used for brewing beer because the sugars ferment into alcohol. Malt and its more processed versions, like malt syrup, add a sweet, caramel-like flavor to foods.

Because barley isn't a common allergen (remember, celiac disease isn't an allergy), it doesn't have to be listed clearly in an ingredients list or in a "CONTAINS" statement on a food label. That means to find sources of barley (and its gluten), you need to know what you are looking for.

def•i•ni•tion

Malt is the term for grain that has been soaked and sprouted. This process brings out the natural sugars in a grain, making malt a great sweetener and flavoring component in many foods, from packaged granola and flavored rice cakes to ice cream and candy. Legally, the use of the term "malt" means it is made from barley. If the malt is made from another grain, such as corn, the label must specify this, as in "corn malt."

Some products say they contain barley right on the label. One common source is vegetable beef soup, which uses barley grains, but many processed foods contain malt or malt flavoring (and may not specifically state barley in the ingredients list), such as malt vinegar, malted milk, hot malt cereal, and ready-to-eat cold cereal. Consider any food off limits because of barley if the label lists any of the following ingredients:

◆ barley

◆ pearl barley

◆ barley malt

◆ barley groats

◆ malt

◆ malt extract

◆ malt flavoring

◆ malt syrup

Read the Label

The names of food additives can be confusing. You know to avoid foods containing malt or malt syrup, so you would think "maltodextrin," a common food ingredient, would also be off limits. However, the use of the prefix "malto" actually has nothing to do with barley. In the United States, maltodextrin is usually made from corn, so this additive should be okay for people who can't eat gluten (and if it was made from wheat, it would have to say so on the label). For more on ingredients you can and can't eat, see Chapters 6 and 7.

So go ahead and try it. Grab a box, a can, or a bottle out of your own pantry, and take a good look. You're an ace label-reader now, but keep reading for more detailed information about how, sometimes, hidden gluten can sneak into your diet. Chapter 5 will help you catch it before it catches you.

The Least You Need to Know

◆ The FDA regulates most of the food we eat (except meat, poultry, and eggs, which the USDA regulates), and makes laws about how those foods can be labeled.

◆ The Food Allergen Labeling and Consumer Protection Act (also known as FALCPA), in force since January 2006, requires that all packaged food labels clearly list the presence of eight major food allergens, including wheat, making it much easier to identify products that contain wheat.

◆ Manufacturers must clearly list major allergens in the ingredients list or in a "CONTAINS" statement right under or next to the ingredients list.

◆ Products that contain rye, barley, and malt also contain gluten but don't have to be quite so clear about it, so people who are gluten-intolerant must read the labels and know what words to look for.

Chapter 5

Hidden Gluten

In This Chapter

◆ Discovering where gluten might be hiding

◆ Avoiding cross-contamination

◆ All about oats

◆ Deciphering food ingredients on the label

Don't look now. Don't panic. And whatever you do, don't turn around. But there's something … evil … creeping … up … behind … you … BOO!

Now, now, don't scream; it's okay; we're sorry; we didn't mean to scare you. In fact, the title of this chapter isn't meant to scare you, either, even though it sounds a little bit like gluten lurks in the shadows of your dinner plate, ready to spring into your mouth without warning.

But you do need to know about hidden glutens. One great thing to know is that recent changes in the law have largely brought gluten out of the closet. Now that wheat must be listed on all packaged food labels regulated by the FDA (see Chapter 4), you can "out" many sources of gluten just by reading the label. But gluten can be in some other sneaky places, too, like your bowl of oatmeal or your prescription medication.

So can you eat it or not? That very confusion is the purpose for this chapter. We're here to clear it up—at least as much as possible. We'll help you decide for yourself whether those gray areas are worth the risk for you by giving you all the available information.

Sniffing Out the Gluten

Sometimes, reading about gluten-free eating, especially on the Internet or in outdated books, can be more confusing than helpful. You may finish an article with more questions than you had when you started reading.

Maybe you've been wondering or worrying about some of the following, because of things you've read or heard:

◆ If a food has just a trace of gluten, is that okay?

◆ What if your food touched food with gluten? Can you still eat it?

◆ Can you get sick from eating food prepared in a pan that prepared something made from gluten or stirred with a spoon or flipped with a spatula that stirred or flipped food containing gluten?

◆ Can you kiss your sweetie after he's/she's just had a big swig of beer or munched on some birthday cake?

◆ What are the nonwheat sources of gluten in food ingredients? How do you know if those ingredients contain gluten?

◆ Are you telling me I can't have my bowl of oatmeal? Is it true? Do oats contain gluten?

◆ Is there ever a case that a food can contain gluten from wheat without disclosing it?

◆ What about soy sauce, smoke flavoring, tamari and shoyu, and other dark, sweetish sauces? If they don't say they contain wheat, are they okay? Or is malted barley hidden in there?

◆ Is caramel color okay? What about other natural or artificial coloring?

◆ What about natural and artificial flavorings or foods that just list "flavoring" on the label?

◆ What about modified food starch and other starch that doesn't specify what it is made from?

◆ Is it true that gluten-containing starch could be in my medication? How do I find out?

◆ What about sweeteners like dextrose, maltose, and glucose syrup?

◆ What about dextrin? I've heard it could contain gluten.

◆ What about hydrolyzed vegetable protein?

Now, never fear; we are here to answer *all* your questions about hidden gluten. So let's tackle these questions one at a time.

A Trace of Gluten: Okay or No Way?

If a food has just a trace of gluten, is that okay?

It can be so tempting … a food might have just a *little* bit of gluten, but you *really* want to eat it. Maybe the very last ingredient on the label is malt. Maybe that piece of chicken is just very lightly dusted in flour. Is that really going to be so very much gluten? Is a *little* bit of gluten okay? Will such a tiny amount really hurt you?

It all depends on what you mean by a *little bit of gluten*. The FDA is currently proposing to allow some foods containing less than 20 parts per million (ppm) of gluten to carry the label "gluten-free." This is a very small amount! But, yes, even if malt is the last ingredient, even if the chicken is just very lightly dusted with flour, even if your salad has just one crouton or you take even one bite of pasta, yes, that could make you sick and injure your body.

Read the Label

Even foods that are labeled "gluten-free" could have traces of gluten. As of this printing, the FDA is still considering the labeling requirements for the use of the term "gluten-free," so check out their website for the most updated information: www.cfsan.fda.gov/~lrd/fr070123.html. Most manufacturers of gluten-free products are responsible, ethical food producers who really want to help those who can't eat gluten. You can probably trust most of their gluten-free claims, but until that term is officially regulated, it's an honor system.

If the food contains even a little wheat, rye, barley, or oats (unless gluten-free variety), then yes, even a little bit could hurt you. If the food contains malted barley, malt, or malt syrup, then yes, even a little bit could hurt you.

Cross-Contamination?

What if your food touched food with gluten? Can you still eat it?

Can you get sick from eating food prepared in a pan that prepared something made from gluten or stirred with a spoon or flipped with a spatula that stirred or flipped food containing gluten?

Can you kiss your sweetie after he's/she's just had a big swig of beer or munched on some birthday cake?

We're lumping all the above questions together because they all deal with a single, very important issue for anyone who can't eat gluten: *cross-contamination*.

def•i•ni•tion

Cross-contamination means that a food that doesn't contain gluten gets contaminated by gluten when it touches a food with gluten or is cooked on a surface that cooked gluten.

You can take a perfectly lovely gluten-free meal and ruin it by cross-contamination. These examples show how this could happen:

◆ **Gluten-free food touching food with gluten.** If you pile up your gluten-free dinner rolls on the plate with the other dinner rolls, the ones touching the gluten rolls will be contaminated. Taking the hamburger off the bun and eating it counts, too. If it was on the bun, it has gluten on it. Those proteins stick to stuff!

Fearless Eater

I ordered a salad in a restaurant the other day and forgot to say "Hold the croutons." So, of course, they brought the salad with croutons. "Oh, no!" I said as the waitress set it before me. "Croutons!" I knew it was my fault, and I was really embarrassed to be a pain, but I had to say, "I'm very sorry; I need a new salad." It's true—if you have croutons on your salad, you can't just pick them off and eat the salad if you want your salad to be gluten-free. This is just one more form of cross-contamination. I know, it's a royal pain, but it's one of the realities of gluten-free eating. Remember to say "skip the croutons," or you'll have to go through what I did. (My waitress was very nice about it, and I apologized. She didn't even roll her eyes ... at least not when I was looking!)

◆ **Cooking gluten-free food in a pan just used to cook a food with gluten.** Some examples might be cooking your plain chicken breast or piece of fish in a pan that you just used to cook a chicken breast or piece of fish covered in breading made with wheat flour or wheat breadcrumbs; cooking your gluten-free pancakes in a pan with the regular pancakes; cooking gluten-free gravy in a pan that just cooked … well, you get the idea.

Some people eating gluten-free thoroughly wash cookware that has cooked food with gluten before using it. Others choose to have separate cookware for gluten-full and gluten-free foods. And still others cook the gluten-free version of the meal first. The choice is up to you, but be sure to do one or the other.

◆ **Sharing utensils.** Use a different spatula, one that hasn't touched gluten, to flip the gluten-free pancakes or remove the gluten-free cookies from the cookie sheet, spoon to stir the gluten-free gravy, or strainer to drain the gluten-free pasta.

◆ **Sharing jars, butter, etc.** Hey, you got your toast crumbs in my peanut butter! People who can't eat gluten are often faced with crumby butter, peanut butter, jam, and other condiments. Either get the squeeze-bottle varieties, or get your own butter, peanut butter, and jam. Label it the "no crumb jar"! You also could institute a "no double-dipping" rule.

◆ **Boiling anything in water that just boiled something with gluten, such as spaghetti or dumplings made with wheat.** If you are making spaghetti for everybody (for example), boil your gluten-free pasta first. Scoop it out, then boil the gluten-filled stuff.

◆ **Putting food with gluten on a plate, then taking it off and putting gluten-free food on the plate.** So you accidentally put the wrong chicken nuggets on your child's plate? Wash the plate. Or use a new plate. (You didn't bake the gluten-free nuggets in the same pan with the gluten-full nuggets, did you?)

◆ **Buying a gluten-free product that was manufactured in a facility that also manufactures products containing wheat.** This one can be confusing. Some products say "gluten-free," but they also say "manufactured in a facility that also manufactures wheat-containing products." If given the choice, some people will choose to eat only products manufactured in a dedicated gluten-free facility, limiting as this can be. Many others trust the manufacturer to clean the equipment sufficiently, as they are required to do.

◆ **Kissing.** Okay, here's the deal. A peck on the cheek or even on the lips probably won't hurt unless the person you are kissing is *really* sloppy and has crumbs all over his or her lips. Wait until he's done chewing that pie to kiss good-bye. It only makes sense—if you can't even eat a piece of salad that a crouton touched, why would you want to put your mouth on somebody chowing down on gluten?

If you're going to get a little more serious about your kissing, your sweetie should brush his or her teeth first. He or she shouldn't mind—who wants his or her kisses to make someone sick?

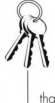

Good for You _____

Food manufacturing facilities get inspected periodically to make sure they are following good manufacturing practices, including proper cleaning of equipment, and most companies do what they are supposed to do. This is one of those cases where you will have to make up your own mind whether or not to eat a product that doesn't contain wheat, rye, or barley, although it was manufactured in a facility that also manufactures wheat. It's *probably* fine, and that's good enough for many people but not for others.

Wheat: No. Gluten: Yes.

What are the nonwheat sources of gluten in food additives? How do you know if those ingredients contain gluten?

As we've mentioned before, the new law requiring food labels to disclose the presence of wheat has been *really helpful* for people who have to eat gluten-free. However, as you should already know by now, wheat isn't the only source of gluten. If a product contains rye, barley, malt, or oats that aren't guaranteed gluten-free, the product has gluten.

If a product contains rye, barley, malt, or oats, in most cases, it has to say so just because products have to reveal their ingredients. However, some ingredients, like flavoring, could be made with these grains and not necessarily say so. This is mostly a problem with malt and most relevant for two food ingredients you often will see: flavorings (natural or artificial) and caramel color.

Barley malt can be used as a flavoring and listed on the label as barley malt or as "flavoring." However, in most cases barley malt will be listed as barley malt on the food label. However, if you are concerned that a flavoring in a product contains barley malt, you could call the manufacturer and ask or just avoid the product.

Caramel color also may be made from malt syrup, but surveys of U.S. manufacturers (originally conducted by *Gluten-Free Living* magazine) indicate that corn is generally used. Of course, because they *could*, it's possible that they *might*, but chances are pretty good that caramel color manufactured in the United States is just fine.

So, unfortunately, what this question boils down to is that the situation with flavorings and caramel color isn't black-and-white, yes-or-no. We realize that, and we're very sorry! But it's the reality of the situation. Here's the lowdown, however:

1. If a product lists "flavoring," "natural flavoring," or "artificial flavoring" on the label and doesn't say what the flavoring is, it probably doesn't contain malted barley … but it could. You'll have to decide if you want to risk it or not, or just call the manufacturer to find out.

2. If a product lists "caramel" or "caramel color" on the label and is made in the United States, chances are very good that it does *not* contain gluten because it is probably made from corn. If the product is made in another country, however, it might be more likely to contain gluten. However, if it was made from wheat, it would still have to say so on the label.

Sowing Your Oats

Are you telling me I can't have my bowl of oatmeal? Is it true? Do oats contain gluten?

Oats, in and of themselves, don't contain gluten. A few studies have found that a small number of individuals have an immunological response to a protein, called avenin, in oats, but most people with celiac disease don't react to this particular protein.

Sadly for oatmeal lovers, however, oats and oat products, including oatmeal and oat flour manufactured in the United States, most likely are contaminated by gluten, either in the field, during harvest, during transport, and/or during processing. Your co-author, Tricia, did a study about this, published in the *New England Journal of Medicine* (Vol 351:2021-2022, November 4, 2004), testing three major brands of oats and oatmeal. She found they all contained gluten.

A couple of companies, however, grow and process oatmeal in gluten-free conditions. If you need your oatmeal, purchase it from them. (Find out more about these companies in Chapter 9.) Many scientific studies conducted over the past 12 years have found that the consumption of moderate amounts of oats known to be gluten-free is safe for most people with celiac disease.

Can They Hide Wheat?

Is there ever a case that a food can contain gluten from wheat without disclosing it?

FDA-regulated products *cannot* hide wheat. However, USDA-regulated products, like meat, poultry, and eggs, aren't required by law to say so if some of the ingredients in the product are derived from wheat, barley, or rye. USDA products do have to list their ingredients, and in most cases, will list wheat, barley, or other gluten-containing ingredients. However, some ingredients on USDA-regulated products could contain wheat, barley, or malt as a subingredient. For meat, poultry, and egg products, any of the following could potentially contain gluten (although they probably don't; in the United States all of these ingredients are likely derived from corn): modified food starch, dextrin, caramel, and glucose syrup. However, if a product contains flavorings made from a protein source, that protein source should be declared on the label. That's good news, since people who are gluten-intolerant react to the proteins in wheat, rye, and barley.

Also, the USDA does expect manufacturers to disclose allergens in any product, so they *should* say if they contain wheat. It's just that so far, the wording of the regulation is a little more ambiguous than the wording of FDA's FALCPA. That may change soon, so keep an ear out, or an eye on this website: www.usda.gov.

Fearless Eater

I was so happy eating my favorite Cobb salad at a local restaurant until I heard that blue cheese contains gluten. You'll see this often mentioned on gluten-free websites as a no-no because the mold used to make those blue streaks is a penicillium culture that could be grown on wheat bread. But wait! Blue cheese *could* be okay. Under FALCPA, if wheat protein was present in the penicillium culture it would have to be declared on the food label. In addition, if wheat protein was present in an incidental additive, such as a processing aid (in this case wheat used to grow the penicillium culture), it must be declared on the label. So read the label. If it doesn't say "wheat," you should be fine. In a restaurant, if you can't see the label, you may decide to skip it.

Getting Sauced

What about soy sauce, smoke flavoring, tamari, shoyu, and other dark, sweetish savory sauces? If they don't say they contain wheat, are they okay? Or is malted barley hidden in there?

Many sauces, particularly Asian sauces like soy sauce and teriyaki sauce, *do* contain wheat, but they are required to say this on the label. It is *possible* that a sauce that lists "flavorings" in the ingredients list contains barley, but chances are, it doesn't.

Although traditionally made tamari is not supposed to contain wheat according to its pure and classic formula, many brands contain wheat and/or barley in some form, so always read the label. When properly formulated, tamari makes a great gluten-free alternative to conventional soy sauce.

The Color of Gluten

Is caramel color okay? What about other natural or artificial coloring?

Caramel color is usually fine, as we mentioned before, if it is made in the United States. Most if not all caramel color in this country is made from corn. However, caramel color *could* be made from wheat starch hydrolysates or barley. If it was made from wheat, it would have to say this on the label. And it probably isn't made from barley. You need not worry about it—at least, we don't.

Other coloring would not contain gluten unless it stated that it contained wheat, so other coloring should be gluten-free, natural or artificial.

Selecting Starches

What about modified food starch and other starch that doesn't specify what it is made from?

If a label lists "starch," it has to be made from corn, by law. Modified food starch is probably made from corn, too, if it is made in the United States. It *could* be made from wheat, but if it is, the label would have to say so, according to the FDA. If it doesn't say "wheat," it should be fine.

Bad Medicine

Is it true that gluten-containing starch could be in my medication? How do I find out?

It is true. Any starch containing wheat has to be disclosed on a food label or nutritional supplement label, but not on a pharmaceutical label, for either over-the-counter or prescription medicine. Just to be sure your medicine is gluten-free, ask your pharmacist to find out, or call the company yourself. If your medication does contain gluten, your doctor should be able to prescribe something else comparable that is gluten-free.

For an excellent article on medications and celiac disease, see "Medications and Celiac Disease-Tips from a Pharmacist" by Steven Plogsted available at: www.healthsystem. virginia.edu/internet/digestive-health/nutritionarticles/plogstedarticle.pdf.

Oh My Sweet!

What about sweeteners like dextrose and maltose? What about glucose syrup? What about dextrin?

First, let's consider dextrose and maltose. Dextrose is glucose, a *monosaccharide*, meaning it contains one unit of sugar. Maltose is a *disaccharide*, meaning it contains two units of sugar. Both can be *hydrolyzed* from starch, but they are both unlikely to contain much in the way of residual protein (that includes gluten) because they are so highly purified. Also, according to the Sugar Association, they are most likely to be made from corn starch in the United States. That means dextrose and maltose should be just fine.

Next, let's consider glucose syrup. This product is less hydrolyzed (processed) than dextrose or maltose, so if it is made from wheat, it could have a greater chance of containing some gluten protein. However, if this were the case, wheat would be listed on the ingredient label. While glucose syrup could be made from a variety of starches, it is typically made from corn starch in the United States. In fact, according to the Code of Federal Regulations, corn syrup sometimes is called glucose syrup. So unless it says "wheat" on the ingredients label, glucose syrup should be fine.

Finally, consider dextrin. While this could be made from wheat and could contain some protein because it isn't completely hydrolyzed, it would have to specify this on the food label if that protein came from wheat. As long as the label doesn't say wheat, dextrin is okay, too.

What all this means to you is that although these ingredients could be made from wheat starch, and may or may not contain any remaining protein/gluten after being broken down into sweeteners (depending on the type of sweetener and the degree of hydrolysis), the label will have to say if the starch came from wheat (in an FDA-regulated product). If it doesn't, it probably came from corn, and you don't have to worry about it.

Hydrolyzed Vegetable Protein

According to FDA regulation, if a hydrolyzed vegetable protein is made from wheat, it has to say "hydrolyzed wheat gluten" or "hydrolyzed wheat protein," or something similarly clear. The FDA says "The names 'hydrolyzed vegetable protein' and 'hydrolyzed protein' are not acceptable because they do not identify the food source of the protein."

Fearless Eater

I ordered some Chinese take-out the other day, and with it came those little packets of soy sauce. I looked at the ingredients list to see if they contained wheat, like most soy sauce does. The packet didn't list wheat, but it did list "hydrolyzed vegetable protein." Now, I know my FDA regulations. I know for a fact that they *aren't allowed to say that.* But they did. Sometimes this happens. If you run into a product that isn't following FDA regulations, it's a good idea to avoid it. That hydrolyzed vegetable protein very well might have been made from wheat. Or maybe not, but if they aren't following the rules, I'm not going to take a risk. You probably wouldn't want to, either. (I used my La Choy soy sauce. It is gluten-free.)

Okay, we admit it—all this hidden gluten business is complicated, and sometimes there really isn't a clear-cut answer. But in many cases, there is! That answer boils down to: look for the words wheat, barley, rye, oats (unless gluten-free variety) or malt.

Now you know the facts as well as we do, so for those few remaining ingredients that might have gluten and might not, you can make a decision for yourself. Knowledge is power!

For more information on all the foods you can and can't eat, listed alphabetically, consult the next two chapters.

The Least You Need to Know

◆ Know where to find gluten: it might be hiding in food ingredients or medications.

◆ Be careful of cross-contamination—don't let other people's gluten get into your food.

◆ Know which sweeteners, sauces, condiments, and other foods have gluten. Always read the label.

Chapter 6

Foods and Ingredients You Can Eat

In This Chapter

◆ All the foods you can eat that are naturally, deliciously gluten-free, listed alphabetically

◆ Explanations for foods and ingredients that might not be familiar

◆ Clarification about some foods and ingredients that are usually gluten-free, but not always, and when to be sure to read the label

When I first started eating gluten-free, I was so confused. I would find something I wanted to eat; I would look at the ingredients label; and well … I just wouldn't be *sure*.

Even though this book gives you some great basic strategies about reading labels and updates on the laws that say packaged FDA-regulated foods have to divulge the presence of wheat in the product, you're probably still worrying about other things. You know the rules, but you look at an ingredients list on something simple on the grocery shelf, like a box of rice mix or a package of bacon, and you just aren't absolutely sure if you can eat it.

I know what I really wanted when I first started eating gluten-free was a list: a definitive, all-encompassing list in one place that I could turn to whenever I needed to know if something was okay to eat. I just wanted it to be *simple*.

Unfortunately, it isn't simple—although it is simpler than it used to be (due to the updated laws). However, a completely definitive list simply isn't possible because there are so many different versions of every food and manufacturers can change their formulas.

So this chapter and the next contain lists—they just aren't *definitive* lists. Instead, they are our best efforts to provide you with information you can use when you go to the grocery store. In this chapter, we list many of the common foods that either almost never have gluten, usually don't have gluten, or are fairly likely to have gluten but don't always.

But please note something very important:

These lists don't exempt you from your duty of reading the label!

We want to make sure you understand that *you must rely on the food label* as the ultimate authority. This list is just a general guideline to help you save time in the store. You'll know that you can go right to the plain fresh fruits and vegetables without worrying about gluten, but you'll also see that you might have to spend more time finding a gluten-free soy sauce or a package of frozen vegetables if they are in a sauce.

To make your browsing easier, we've arranged this chapter in alphabetical order. Next to each item, we've placed a symbol:

☺ This smiley face means the food or ingredient is *almost always gluten-free*. We apply this to fresh plain foods, like bananas and fresh eggs. We don't say *always* because we never know what somebody might do to a food, and we can't possibly know every single scenario for every single food product. But in most cases, these foods are A-OK.

▲ This triangle means the food or ingredient is *usually* gluten-free. Read the label to be sure, but in most cases, you'll see that the food is just fine. (But once again ... *always read the label!*)

⚡ This lightning bolt means beware—this food or ingredient often contains gluten. You can find gluten-free examples if you look, but you'll probably have to look closely, and you may not find anything in your area (although you can order many gluten-free versions of common gluten-filled products online—see Chapter 9 for some of our favorites). You'll also see this symbol in the next chapter, which lists foods you can't eat, i.e., foods that usually or always contain gluten.

Also for your convenience, if a food goes by more than one name, you'll find it in more than one place (such as rice under "R" and white rice under "W" and brown rice under "B"). You will probably read through this book once and maybe refer to certain parts every now and then, but we suspect you'll turn to these two chapters again and again whenever you just want to be sure, or jog your memory, about whether something is okay to eat or not. (Or if you need another reminder to *read the label!* Yes, we say that a lot, but we consider it our gluten-free mantra.)

Note that one thing you *won't* find in this chapter are the products that normally contain gluten but are specifically formulated to be gluten-free, like gluten-free bread, gluten-free pasta, gluten-free cookies, etc. Can you imagine how long the "G" section would be? For the lowdown on gluten-free products (especially some of our personal favorites), check out Chapter 9.

So here you go; here is your master list. If you find things that we haven't listed here, feel free to add your own entries to this book. We won't mind one bit if you cover this chapter with your personal notes.

If an ingredient doesn't specify, we mean the plain, fresh version without added sauces, seasonings, or flavorings.

Read the Label

Did we mention you should never totally trust anybody's list and you should always read the label as the ultimate authority on whether a food is gluten-free? We did mention that? Well, it won't hurt to mention it again.

A

▲   Alcoholic beverages (Distilled liquor, wine, and champagne are gluten-free; regular beer is not. Some alcoholic beverages may contain flavorings added after distillation. If you are concerned about flavorings, contact the manufacturer. For more specific information on alcohol see Chapter 10.)

☺   Almonds, plain, raw

⚡   Almonds, seasoned

☺   Amaranth

☺   Apple cider

☺   Arborio rice, not seasoned

☺   Arrowroot

☺   Artichoke

☺   Artificial sweetener, Nutrasweet, Sweet'N Low, Equal, etc.

☺   Avocado

B

▲   Bacon (Many brands are gluten-free, but check the label to be sure.)

▲   Baked beans (Many varieties are gluten-free, but some types contain gluten, so beware.)

☺   Baker's yeast

☺   Baking powder

☺   Baking soda

☺   Basmati rice, not seasoned

☺   Beans, dried or fresh (Black, red, white, garbanzo, pinto, and green beans, of course … all of 'em are just fine in their dried or plain, fresh state with no sauce or seasoning.)

☺   Bean flour, 100 percent

☺   Beef, plain roast, steak, ground beef, etc.

⚡   Beef, seasoned or sauced

☺   Berries, plain, all types

▲   Berries, sweetened, frozen or canned or in a sauce.

☺   Besan, chickpea flour, 100 percent

▲   Black beans, canned (These sometimes have added seasoning.)

☺   Black beans, dried

▲   Black-eyed peas, canned (These could contain seasoning.)

☺   Black-eyed peas, dried

☺   Black-eyed peas, frozen, unseasoned

▲   Bologna (Many brands are gluten-free, but check the label to be sure.)

⚡   Breakfast cereal (Most brands are made with gluten-containing grains and/or flavored with malt. You can find varieties without gluten in health food stores, but read the label.)

Fearless Eater
Not being a big fan of meat, I rely heavily on beans as a good, delicious, and inexpensive source of gluten-free protein. Dried beans are the most economical, but canned beans (well rinsed to rid them of excess sodium) are much more convenient and not too expensive, either. I look for them on sale and buy a bunch of cans to keep in my pantry all the time. I think a bowl of hot rice with black beans, fresh lime juice, fresh cilantro, and a little chopped, sautéed onion, garlic, and green pepper makes a fine dinner.

▲   Breakfast meats (Many brands are gluten-free, but check the label to be sure.)

☺   Brown rice, plain

⚡   Brown rice, seasoned mixes

☺   Brown rice flour, 100 percent rice

☺   Brown sugar, 100 percent sugar

☺   Buckwheat, 100 percent

☺   Buckwheat groats, 100 percent

⚡   Buckwheat pancake and baking mixes (They often contain wheat flour or malted barley, so look at the label. Some contain 100 percent buckwheat or a combination of gluten-free grains.)

☺   Butter, plain, sweet cream, or salted

☺   Buttermilk

C

⚡   Candy (Many mainstream brands contain wafers, cookies, or malt flavoring, so read the label.)

▲   Canned vegetables (These are okay as long as they don't contain a gluten-containing sauce.)

▲   Caramel color (According to the Code of Federal Regulations, caramel color *can* be made from malt syrup or starch hydrolysates, but is generally made from corn in the United States.)

⚡   Carob chips (Some varieties include malt, so choose carefully.)

▲ Carob powder (Look for varieties that are 100 percent carob powder and are gluten-free.)

☺ Cashews, plain

⚡ Cashews, seasoned

☺ Cassava, another name for tapioca starch

⚡ Cereal, breakfast (Look for cereal containing rice, corn, or other nongluten grains and *not* flavored with malt. This excludes most mainstream brands. Also look in your health food or specialty store for gluten-free options.)

▲ Cheese, natural or processed (Some cheeses could contain modified food starch from wheat (ricotta) or cultures grown on wheat (blue cheese), so check the label. Processed cheese spreads and sauces could also contain gluten.)

⚡ Cheese sauce (This is often thickened with gluten-containing ingredients, so proceed with caution.)

☺ Chestnuts

☺ Chickpeas, canned, 100 percent water-packed, no seasoning

☺ Chickpeas, dried

☺ Chickpea flour, 100 percent chickpeas

☺ Chicken, plain

⚡ Chicken, seasoned or sauced

Good for You _____

Just one more reason to buy organic and/or free-range poultry: these minimally processed meats are much less likely to be injected with high-sodium "basting solution," which may or may not contain gluten. Even if it doesn't contain gluten, basting solution probably contains chemicals and preservatives, ingredients you are probably better off without.

▲ Chocolate (It could contain malt flavoring or other added ingredients, so check. Gourmet dark chocolate bars are often okay, but read the label to be sure.)

☺ Cider, apple or pear

☺ Citrus fruits, fresh oranges, lemons, limes, grapefruit, etc.

☺ Citrus juice, orange, lemon, lime, grapefruit, etc., 100 percent juice

☺ Converted rice, parboiled rice, 100 percent

⚡ Converted rice mixes with seasoning

☺ Cocoa for baking, 100 percent only

▲ Cocoa mix, hot chocolate mix (Some brands are gluten-free, but others contain gluten, so read the label.)

▲ Coconut, packaged, sweetened or unsweetened

☺ Coconut, raw, fresh

☺ Coffee, 100 percent, beans or ground, brewed or instant

▲ Coffee, flavored, instant mixes

☺ Confectioners' sugar

▲ Cooking oil, flavored or seasoned

☺ Cooking oil, 100 percent plain, all types

▲ Corn, canned or frozen (Some versions have seasoning or sauce, but 100 percent water-packed is fine.)

☺ Corn, fresh, plain

☺ Corn bran, 100 percent

▲ Corn chips, flavored (Seasoning could contain gluten.)

☺ Corn chips, plain, unflavored

⚡ Corn flakes cereal (Most brands are flavored with malt.)

☺ Corn flour, 100 percent

☺ Corn gluten (This kind of gluten does not bother people with celiac disease.)

▲ Corn grits (Some packaged varieties contain gluten.)

☺ Corn malt

☺ Corn starch, 100 percent

☺ Corn syrup

▲ Corn tortillas (These are almost always gluten-free, but check the label.)

▲ Corned beef (Many brands are gluten-free, but check the label to be sure.)

☺ Cornmeal, 100 percent

▲ Cottage cheese (Lower-fat varieties often contain filler so check the label carefully.)

☺ Cream, plain

▲ Cream cheese, flavored (Lower-fat varieties often contain filler so check the label carefully.)

▲ Cream cheese, plain

☺ Cream of Tartar

▲ Creamer, nondairy creamer

 Good for You _____

Non-dairy creamer often contains trans fat (hydrogenated or partially hydrogenated oil). Choose products that are both gluten- and trans fat-free.

D

⚡ Dates (Many varieties are powdered to prevent sticking, and the powder may be a gluten-containing flour, like oat flour.)

▲ Deli meat (Many brands are gluten-free, but check the label, or ask the person behind the deli counter to check it or let you see the ingredients list on the package.)

▲ Dextrin (As long as it just says "dextrin," it is gluten-free. If the dextrin is made from wheat, the label will state this on an FDA-regulated product.)

▲ Distilled liquor (All pure distilled alcohol, such as vodka, gin, rum, whiskey, and Scotch, is gluten-free. Some alcohols may have flavorings added after distillation. If you are concerned about flavorings contact the manufacturer.)

▲ Distilled vinegar (Plain distilled vinegar is always gluten-free as are the fermented vinegars cider, wine, and balsamic. Malt vinegar is not gluten-free, and flavored vinegars could contain gluten.)

▲ Dried fruit (Most dried fruit should be fine, except dates with gluten-containing flour.)

Read the Label

We've seen dates dusted with oat flour, which means they contain gluten. Why do they dust dates with oat flour? So they don't stick together, I suppose. If you want to eat dates, look for undusted varieties, or those dusted with sugar.

E

▲   Edamame, dried snacks (These may contain gluten.)

☺   Edamame, plain, soybeans

☺   Eggs, fresh

▲   Egg substitute

☺   Equal, artificial sweetener

F

▲   Fava beans, canned or frozen (Beans are gluten-free if water-packed, but some versions contain added seasoning and possibly gluten.)

☺   Fava beans, dried

☺   Fish, fresh, without seasoning or sauce

⚡   Fish in breading, seasoning, or sauce (See Chapter 9 for my favorite gluten-free fish sticks!)

☺   Flaxseed, 100 percent

☺   Flaxseed oil, 100 percent

▲   Frosting (Many are okay, but some flavors and brands could contain malt.)

▲   Frozen yogurt (Some contain gluten-filled ingredients like cookie pieces, and some brands are flavored with malt.)

▲   Fruit, canned or frozen (Always gluten-free if water-packed.)

☺   Fruit, fresh, plain

☺   Fruit jam or jelly

☺ Fruit juice, 100 percent fruit

▲ Fruit-flavored beverages

G

☺ Garbanzo bean flour, 100 percent

▲ Garbanzo beans, canned (Always gluten-free if water-packed.)

☺ Garbanzo beans, dried

▲ Gelatin, flavored/sweetened

☺ Gelatin, plain, 100 percent

☺ Gin

☺ Glutinous rice (This sounds like gluten, but it isn't.)

☺ Glutinous rice flour, 100 percent

▲ Green peas, canned or frozen (Always gluten-free if water-packed.)

☺ Green peas, fresh

⚡ Green peas, seasoned or sauced

▲ Grits, corn or hominy, flavored

☺ Grits, corn or hominy, plain, 100 percent

☺ Ground beef, plain

⚡ Ground beef, seasoned

H

☺ Half-and-half, plain

▲ Ham (Many brands are gluten-free, but check the label.)

▲ Hard candy (Some could be flavored with malt or contain filling with gluten-containing ingredients.)

☺ Hazelnuts, plain

⚡ Hazelnuts, seasoned

> **Fearless Eater**
>
> I recently discovered Hazelnut Milk, made by Pacific. It's delicious on hot rice cereal (I add some walnuts and blueberries or raisins), and it's gluten-free.

☺   Herbs, pure single-herb

▲   Herb mixes (Mixes that contain 100 percent herbs are fine, but some contain other ingredients and possibly wheat starch.)

☺   High-fructose corn syrup

☺   Honey, 100 percent

▲   Hot rice cereal, plain (Be sure it isn't flavored with malt.)

I

⚡   Ice cream (Some contain gluten-filled additives like cookie or brownie pieces, binders containing gluten, or malt flavoring. Look for brand with just a few basic ingredients, like milk, cream, sugar, egg yolks, and vanilla.)

▲   Icing (Check the label to be sure these aren't flavored with malt.)

▲   Instant coffee (Plain is fine, but some flavored varieties could contain gluten.)

☺   Instant rice, plain

⚡   Instant rice mixes (These often contain gluten! Look carefully.)

J

☺   Jam

▲   Jasmine rice, flavored or seasoned

☺   Jasmine rice, plain

☺   Jelly

☺   Juice, 100 percent fruit

▲   Juice drink

K

▲ Kasha, roasted buckwheat (This is fine if 100 percent buckwheat, but read the label to be sure there aren't added ingredients.)

▲ Ketchup (Usually okay, but check the label just in case.)

L

▲ Legumes, frozen or canned (Always gluten-free if water-packed.)

☺ Legumes, plain, dried or fresh

⚡ Lentil soup (Mainstream varieties often contain gluten.)

☺ Lentils, plain

▲ Liqueur (Flavorings may be added after distillation. If you are concerned about flavoring ingredients in liqueur, contact the manufacturer)

☺ Long-grain rice, 100 percent, plain

⚡ Long-grain rice seasoned mixes

▲ Luncheon meats, bologna, salami, smoked turkey, deli ham (Many brands are gluten-free, but check the label.)

M

▲ Maltodextrin

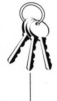

Good for You _____

Maltodextrin sounds like it has gluten because of that deceiving "malto" in the word, but it's almost always gluten-free. According to the Code of Federal Regulations, maltodextrin can be made from corn, rice, or potato starch. If it is made from wheat, the label will say so.

☺ Maple syrup, 100 percent

▲ Maple-flavored syrup

☺ Margarine, 100 percent

☺ Marmalade, 100 percent fruit and sugar or corn syrup

☺ Meat, fresh, plain

⚡ Meat, seasoned, flavored, or in sauce

☺ Milk, plain, not sweetened or flavored

▲ Milk, flavored, chocolate, vanilla, banana, etc. (Malted milk *always* contains gluten.)

▲ Milk, nut—such as almond or hazelnut milk (Some brands contain wheat or barley.)

▲ Milk, rice (Some brands contain wheat or barley.)

▲ Milk, soy (Some brands contain wheat or barley.)

☺ Millet, plain, 100 percent

☺ Mixed nuts, plain

⚡ Mixed nuts, seasoned

☺ Modified corn starch

▲ Modified food starch (Modified food starch may be made from a variety of grains, including wheat. However, if it is made from wheat, it will be stated on the label. If the label does not include the word "wheat," the modified food starch in that product is gluten-free in an FDA-regulated food product.)

☺ Molasses, 100 percent

▲ Mustard, flavored, brown, grainy, etc.

☺ Mustard, plain yellow

N

▲ Nondairy creamer (Choose gluten-free and trans fat-free varieties.)

▲ Nondairy whipped topping

▲ Nut butter (100 percent nut butter is always gluten-free, but some varieties may contain added ingredients.)

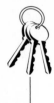

Good for You _____

If you miss peanut butter and jelly sandwiches (or almond butter and marmalade sandwiches, like I miss!) and you can't find any gluten-free bread you love (although check out Chapter 9 for some ideas), just put that nut butter and fruit spread on a gluten-free rice cake, or make mini sandwiches between gluten-free rice crackers. In my opinion, that rice-cake crunch just adds to the gastronomic satisfaction.

☺ Nut flour, 100 percent nuts

▲ Nut flour mixes

▲ Nut milk (Some brands contain wheat or barley.)

☺ Nutrasweet, sweetener

☺ Nuts, raw, plain, unflavored

⚡ Nuts, seasoned or flavored, like tamari almonds, nut mixes

O

☺ Oil, 100 percent, all types

☺ Olive oil, plain, unflavored, 100 percent

▲ Olives, flavored or stuffed

☺ Olives, green, black, etc., plain

P

☺ Parboiled rice, converted rice, plain

⚡ Parboiled rice, converted rice, seasoned mixes

▲ Peanut butter (100 percent peanut varieties are fine, but many brands contain added ingredients.)

⚡ Peanuts, flavored

☺ Peanuts, plain, boiled or roasted, without added ingredients

☺ Peas, fresh, plain

▲ Peas, frozen or canned (Always gluten-free if water-packed.)

⚡ Peas, seasoned or sauced

☺ Pecans, plain

⚡ Pecans, seasoned

☺ Pepper, 100 percent, black, white, red, green, etc.

▲ Pepper-based seasoning mix

▲ Pickle relish

▲ Pickled vegetables

▲ Pickles, dill, sweet, bread-and-butter, kosher, etc.

▲ Pinto beans, canned (Water-packed will be gluten-free, but some varieties contain other ingredients.)

☺ Pinto beans, dried

▲ Pinto beans, refried

▲ Pinto beans, seasoned or flavored

▲ Popcorn, flavored

☺ Popcorn, plain

Good for You _____

Some of your culinary traditions may need to change, but popcorn while you watch a movie? No problem. Believe it or not, popcorn is a whole grain and full of fiber. Just make sure to go easy on the butter and salt.

▲ Pork, cured, bacon, sausage, ham, etc.

☺ Pork, plain

⚡ Pork, seasoned or sauced

▲ Pork products

▲ Pork-and-beans, canned

☺ Potato, white and sweet, plain

▲ Potatoes, flavored

▲   Potatoes, instant

☺   Potato chips, plain

▲   Potato chips, seasoned or flavored

☺   Potato flour, 100 percent

☺   Potato starch, 100 percent

☺   Poultry, fresh, plain

⚡   Poultry, seasoned or in sauce

☺   Powdered sugar

▲   Processed cheese, American cheese or Velveeta

Q

☺   Quinoa, 100 percent

☺   Quinoa pasta, 100 percent quinoa

▲   Quinoa pasta, blended with other grains

R

☺   Raw nuts, plain

☺   Rice, plain, unseasoned, white, brown, wild … go crazy!

☺   Rice bran, 100 percent

▲   Rice cereal, hot (Be sure it is 100 percent rice and not flavored with malt.)

▲   Rice milk (Some brands contain wheat or barley.)

⚡   Rice mixes (Many mainstream brands contain gluten.)

☺   Rice noodles, 100 percent rice

☺   Rice pasta, 100 percent rice

▲   Risotto (Some risotto mixes contain gluten; others don't.)

☺   Rum

S

▲ Salad dressing (Some brands contain gluten; some don't. Read the label or make it from scratch.)

▲ Salami (Many brands are gluten-free, but check the label.)

☺ Salmon, plain, without seasoning or sauce

⚡ Salmon, seasoned or in sauce

▲ Salsa (Most are fine, but at least one brand contains barley malt, so check the label.)

☺ Sashimi, plain

☺ Sauerkraut, plain

▲ Sausage (Many brands are gluten-free, but check the label.)

☺ Scotch

⚡ Seafood, in sauce, seasoned, or breaded (Breaded in 100 percent cornmeal is okay.)

☺ Seafood, plain, without seasoning, sauce, or breading

☺ Seed flour, 100 percent seeds, such as from sesame

☺ Seeds, plain, sesame, sunflower, pumpkin, etc.

⚡ Seeds, seasoned

☺ Sesame butter, tahini, plain

☺ Sesame seeds, plain

▲ Sherbet

☺ Short-grain rice, plain

⚡ Short-grain seasoned rice mixes

Fearless Eater

I've started sprinkling sesame seeds where I never thought of sprinkling sesame seeds before—into hot rice cereal, on top of salad, mixed into plain yogurt with a spoonful of molasses, on top of gluten-free pancakes, in gluten-free cookie batter, even as a garnish on soup. Roast them for a few minutes in a dry heavy skillet to bring out the flavor.

☺ Shortening, plain

☺ Shrimp, plain, unseasoned, not breaded

⚡ Shrimp, seasoned, sauced, or breaded (Breaded in 100 percent cornmeal is fine.)

▲ Smoked meat (Many brands are gluten-free, but check the label.)

▲ Soba noodles (Look for 100 percent buckwheat varieties, not the kind that also contain wheat.)

▲ Soft drinks, regular and diet (These are probably okay, but check the label.)

☺ Sorghum, a gluten-free grain

⚡ Soup, canned (Many varieties contain gluten.)

☺ Soy, 100 percent

▲ Soy milk (Some varieties contain barley malt or wheat.)

▲ Soy nuts

⚡ Soy products, flavored

⚡ Soy sauce (Most have wheat, but some brands are just fine; read the label.)

☺ Soybeans, plain

▲ Soybeans, seasoned

▲ Spices (Pure 100 percent spices are fine, and most contain only the spice. Spice mixes could contain gluten if they have added ingredients.)

☺ Splenda, an artificial sweetener

▲ Starch (If the label just says "starch," that means cornstarch, and it is gluten-free.)

☺ Steak, plain (But read the label on the steak sauce.)

☺ Sugar, plain, all types, white, brown, raw, confectioner's

▲ Sushi (Avoid the kinds containing "crunch"—bits of fried tempura batter—or those with rice seasoned with soy sauce. All prepackaged deli foods are required to carry a label with ingredients list. Avoid any deli foods without a label.)

☺ Sweet'N Low, an artificial sweetener

☺ Sweet potato, canned, 100 percent sweet potato

☺ Sweet potato, fresh, plain

T

▲ Taco shells (The hard shells are made from corn. The soft shells are often made from flour and have gluten, but you can make soft tacos with corn tortillas, too.)

⚡ Tamari sauce (Traditionally made tamari is supposed to be wheat-free, but many brands contain wheat and/or barley; read the label.)

☺ Tapioca, 100 percent

☺ Taro root, 100 percent

☺ Tea, black, green, white, or herbal, 100 percent tea or herbs

▲ Tea, flavored

☺ Tempeh, plain (flavored varieties often contain wheat)

☺ Tomato paste, plain

▲ Tomato sauce, flavored

☺ Tomato sauce, plain

☺ Tomatoes, canned, stewed, roasted, etc., 100 percent

☺ Tofu, plain (Flavored, baked, and smoked varieties often contain wheat.)

⚡ Tofu burgers, hot dogs, etc. (Most fake meat products, including most of the mainstream brands, contain wheat gluten, but a few brands contain tofu and no gluten, so read the label.)

☺ Tuna, fresh or canned, plain

Good for You _____

Plain tuna doesn't contain gluten, but you might want to choose light over white (albacore) versions. Light tuna is likely to contain less mercury than white tuna.

☺ Turkey, fresh, plain

⚡ Turkey, seasoned, injected with basting solution (like many Thanksgiving turkeys sold in supermarkets), in sauce, or prepared in loaves and packaged

V

☺ Vanilla, pure

☺ Vegetable juice, 100 percent

☺ Vegetable oil, 100 percent

▲ Vegetables, canned, frozen, or in sauce

☺ Vegetables, plain

▲ Vinegar, except for malt and some flavored vinegars

☺ Vodka

W

▲ Wasabi (Pure wasabi is fine, but many pastes and preparations contain added ingredients.)

▲ Whipped cream

▲ Whipped topping

☺ Whiskey

☺ White rice, plain

⚡ White rice, seasoned or mixes

☺ White sugar, 100 percent

☺ Wild rice, plain

⚡ Wild rice mixes

☺ Wine, red, white, or rose, all types

Y

▲ Yogurt, flavored

☺ Yogurt, plain

▲ Yams, canned

☺ Yams, fresh

The Least You Need to Know

◆ The list in this chapter can guide you toward foods that almost always don't contain gluten, usually don't contain gluten, or often contain gluten.

◆ Never rely solely on a list—always read the food label, which is the ultimate authority on whether any particular food is gluten-free.

Chapter 7

Foods and Ingredients You Can't Eat

In This Chapter

- ◆ Alphabetical listing for all the gluten-containing foods you can't eat

- ◆ Explanations for unfamiliar foods and ingredients

- ◆ Clarification about foods and ingredients that usually, but not always, contain gluten

This chapter is the partner to Chapter 6. Here, we list alphabetically (for your convenience) all the foods that either *always* have gluten or *probably* have gluten. Sure, this chapter contains plenty of off-limit foods that we've listed to keep you safe and healthy. But notice that Chapter 6—all the great stuff you *can* eat—is longer.

One thing to keep in mind as you survey this list or use it as your guide while grocery shopping: many items listed here also have gluten-free versions that are just fine. If we list "pasta" or "doughnuts" or "cake" or "chocolate chip cookies," we don't mean the gluten-free varieties. We mean the "standard American" varieties. We didn't want to clutter this list by adding "(except gluten-free types)" after every single entry, so just assume that

that's what we mean. For more information on products specifically formulated to be gluten-free, including some of our favorites, see Chapter 9.

To help make your shopping a little bit easier, we've also labeled the items in this chapter with helpful icons.

▲ As in Chapter 6, a few items carry the triangle symbol. This means the food or ingredient is *usually* gluten-free. Read the label to be sure, but in most cases, you'll see that the food is just fine.

⚡ As in Chapter 6, the lightning bolt symbol means the food or ingredient *often* contains gluten, but there are some gluten-free varieties, if you bother to look. We don't mean food specially formulated to be gluten-free—we talk about this food category in Chapter 9. We just mean that some brands or varieties happen to be gluten-free. We often use soy sauce as an example, and it's a good example, here, too. It usually has gluten, but a few brands don't, so it gets the lightning bolt.

You'll also notice some crossover between this chapter and Chapter 6. We do list a few lightning-bolt items in Chapter 6, just in case you are wondering about them when browsing for okay foods. But those same foods, and some others, are listed here.

⊘ This symbol means the food *always*, or *almost* always, has gluten if made in the conventional manner. This includes things like wheat bread, malt vinegar, and semolina pasta. You can feel confident that you should *not* eat a food or a food containing an ingredient if it carries this symbol.

So when in doubt about an ingredient, look it up here or in Chapter 6. Between these two chapters, you should be able to avoid the bad stuff and find plenty of the good stuff to keep you satisfied. Of course, we can't list every single food and ingredient that exists, but we hope to help you out a lot with these master lists.

And, as always, read the ingredients list of all foods you purchase! That list is always the final authority on whether or not a food contains gluten.

A

▲ Artificial flavoring (If a flavoring contains wheat, it will be declared on the food label. A flavoring could contain barley malt, but this will usually be listed in the ingredients list.)

B

⊘ Bagels

⊘ Baguette

▲ Baked beans (Some have gluten-containing sauce.)

⊘ Barley

⚡ Barley grass, can contain seeds

⚡ Beer (Most beer is made from malted barley, but a few mainstream gluten-free beers are available. For more about these, see Chapter 10.)

⊘ Biscuits (You can buy gluten-free biscuit mixes. See Chapter 9.)

▲ Blue cheese (If the penicillium culture added to the cheese contains wheat protein, wheat should be declared on the label.)

⚡ Bouillon cubes (Many brands contain gluten.)

⊘ Bran, wheat

⊘ Bread, brown (See Chapter 9 for gluten-free versions.)

⊘ Bread, mixed grain (To find gluten-free versions, check out resources in Chapter 9.)

⊘ Bread, rye

⊘ Bread, wheat

⊘ Bread, white (To find gluten-free versions, see resources in Chapter 9.)

⊘ Bread, whole-wheat

Fearless Eater

Ah, bread … it may be the thing you miss the most! After about a week of eating gluten-free, I wanted some bread in the *worst way*. The first few store-bought gluten-free breads I bought were a bust, but I finally found some I thought were just delicious (for those days when I didn't have time to bake my own batch). My two favorites I was able to find in my local grocery store: Ener-G Harvest Loaf and Kinnikinnick Brown Sandwich Bread. Both are at their best when toasted, in my opinion.

⊘   Bread crumbs (To find gluten-free versions, see resources in Chapter 9.)

⊘   Bread flour

⊘   Bread pudding

⊘   Bread stuffing mix

⚡   Breakfast bars, cereal bars, energy bars

⊘   Brownies (See Chapter 9 for gluten-free versions.)

⊘   Bulgur, bulgur wheat

C

⊘   Cake (See Chapter 9 for gluten-free versions.)

⊘   Candy with gluten ingredients like wafers, cookies, pretzels, or "crunch" (Also, many commercial candies are flavored with malt.)

⚡   Cereal, cold breakfast (Most commercial brands contain gluten.)

⚡   Cereal, hot (Many commercial brands contain gluten.)

⊘   Cereal bars (To find gluten-free versions, see resources in Chapter 9.)

⚡   Cheese sauce (Many are thickened with flour, so read the label.)

▲   Cocoa mix (Some contain gluten, others don't.)

⚡   Communion wafers (Almost all contain wheat, although you can purchase a gluten-free variety from Ener-G Foods as well as a low-gluten variety that is acceptable to the Catholic Church. See the sidebar about communion wafers in Chapter 9 for more information about this product.)

⊘   Cookies (But Chapter 9 has specialty gluten-free versions.)

⚡   Cornbread (Most cornbread and cornbread mixes contain wheat flour.)

⊘   Couscous

⚡   Crackers (Some crackers in the grocery store are gluten-free, so check the label.)

⊘   Cream of Wheat hot cereal

⊘   Croissant

⊘   Croutons (But Chapter 9 lists a gluten-free version.)

⊘   Cupcakes, prepackaged snack cakes and mixes

D

○   Dinkle, another name for spelt

○   Doughnuts (But Chapter 9 has a specialty gluten-free version.)

○   Dried wheat gluten

○   Durum, durum wheat

E

○   Eggroll wrappers

○   Einkorn, a variety of wheat

○   Emmer, another name for durum wheat

⚡   Energy bars

F

○   Farina, an instant wheat cereal, also the Italian brand name for Cream of Wheat cereal

○   Farro, another name for spelt, a variety of wheat

▲   Flavoring (If a flavoring contains wheat, wheat will be declared on the food label. A flavoring could contain barley malt, but this will usually be listed in the ingredients list.)

○   Flour, normally wheat flour. (An ingredients list will say "wheat flour," but the front of the package might not, so check the label)

 Read the Label

There are plenty of gluten-free flours that are just fine for you to eat, including rice, potato, buckwheat, teff, tapioca, millet, amaranth, and corn. The source of these flours will generally be named on the front of the packaging. If the front of a package merely says "flour" this is most likely wheat flour but check the ingredients list. If it is wheat flour it will say so.

○   French toast, packaged varieties

G

○   Germ, from a gluten-containing grain

○   Gluten, wheat (obviously)

○   Graham crackers

○   Graham flour

⚡   Gravy (Most are thickened with wheat flour, but some may be thickened with cornstarch.)

▲   Grits (Avoid these if they contain added wheat flour or are flavored with malt. Unflavored 100 percent corn or hominy grits are okay.)

H

○   Hydrolyzed wheat protein

○   Hydrolyzed wheat starch

Read the Label _____

Occasionally, you may see the terms "hydrolyzed plant protein" or "hydrolyzed vegetable protein" in an ingredients list. Technically, this isn't a legal term anymore. The manufacturers have to say what plant or vegetable they use. However, some products slip through the cracks—I've seen the term on soy sauce packets in restaurants. If it doesn't say what the plant or vegetable source is, it could be wheat, so avoid it.

I

○   Ice cream flavored with malt or containing gluten ingredients, like cookie or brownie pieces

⚡   Imitation seafood, like imitation crab, which usually contains wheat

⚡   Instant rice mixes, seasoned (Many but not all contain gluten.)

K

○   Kamut, a variety of wheat

L

◎ Licorice (There are gluten-free varieties available, but the "regular" kind contains gluten.)

M

◎ Macaroni

◎ Malt (Sometimes, malt can be made from corn, but the food label will say. If it just says "malt," it contains gluten.)

◎ Malt extract

◎ Malt flavoring

◎ Malt syrup

◎ Malt vinegar

◎ Malt-o-Meal hot cereal

◎ Malted milk

▲ Marinade (You won't know what's in it unless you read the label.)

◎ Matza, matzo, unleavened wheat bread

◎ Matza flour, matzo flour

◎ Modified food starch, wheat (If wheat is not declared in the ingredients list or Contains statement, the modified food starch is gluten-free in an FDA-regulated product.)

◎ Muffins (But see Chapter 9 for gluten-free resources.)

N

▲ Natural flavoring (If a flavoring contains wheat, wheat will be declared on the food label. A flavoring could contain barley malt, but this will usually be included in the ingredients list.)

⚡ Noodles (Most are made from wheat, semolina, durum, whole-wheat, spinach, etc.)

Good for You _____

Pasta lovers rejoice! You can buy a few absolutely delicious gluten-free pastas made from rice, quinoa, and other nongluten grains. Tricia and I both particularly like the Tinkyada brand, and I'm also a fan of Lundberg Family Farms brand.

O

⚡ Oat bran (For more about oats, see Chapter 5; for gluten-free oat manufacturers, see Chapter 9.)

⚡ Oat fiber (For more about oats, see Chapter 5; for gluten-free oat manufacturers, see Chapter 9.)

⚡ Oatmeal (For more about oats, see Chapter 5; for gluten-free oat manufacturers, see Chapter 9.)

⚡ Oats, instant, old-fashioned, rolled, steel cut (For more about oats, see Chapter 5; for gluten-free oat manufacturers, see Chapter 9.)

⊘ Orzo, pasta shaped like rice

P

⊘ Pancakes (See Chapter 9 for gluten-free mixes.)

⚡ Pasta (Most is made from wheat, semolina, durum, whole wheat, spinach, etc., but gluten-free varieties are made from rice, quinoa, and other nongluten grains.)

⊘ Pastry (Any variety made from wheat flour, including white flour and pastry flour, contains gluten. See Chapter 9 for gluten-free versions.)

⊘ Pearl barley

⊘ Phyllo dough

⊘ Pie crust (Chapter 9 includes resources for finding gluten-free versions.)

⊘ Pizza crust

Good for You _____

Traditional pizza crust may be off the list, but there are some ingenious gluten-free versions, including a rice-crust pizza by Amy's Kitchen, a cheese-based pizza crust made by Van Harden's (a brand made right here in Iowa where I live—www.vanharden.com), and a crustless pizza with a sausage base by Lou Malnati's of Chicago (www.tastesofchicago.com/product/392/4).

- ⊘ Pretzels
- ⊘ Puff pastry

R

- ⚡ Ramen noodles (Most brands are made with wheat noodles, but there are a few "instant noodle bowls" and ramen-like products made with 100 percent rice noodles.)
- ⚡ Rice mixes, seasoned (These often contain gluten.)
- ⊘ Rye
- ⊘ Rye bread
- ⊘ Rye crisp
- ⊘ Rye flour

S

- ⚡ Salad dressing (Many bottled varieties contain gluten.)
- ⚡ Salad "kits" (Many contain croutons, and the dressing in the packet may have gluten. If the dressing label doesn't reveal gluten and you throw out the croutons, these kits are fine as long as the croutons are packaged separately.)
- ⊘ Sauce thickened with wheat flour
- ⚡ Seasoning mixes (These could contain gluten, so read the label.)
- ⊘ Seitan, sometimes called "wheat meat," almost pure wheat gluten
- ⊘ Semolina, a ground durum wheat often used to make pasta

⊘ Shoyu sauce, a variety of soy sauce made with wheat

▲ Soba noodles (These are made from buckwheat, but many also contain some wheat, so read the label.)

⚡ Soup, canned (Many varieties contain gluten, so read the label.)

⚡ Soy sauce (Most varieties contain wheat, although you can find some without wheat, so read the label.)

⊘ Spelt, a variety of wheat

⊘ Sprouted wheat or barley

⊘ Stuffing mix (bread)

T

⊘ Tabbouleh salad, deli or mix

Fearless Eater

I was pleased to discover that I could make a really good faux tabbouleh salad using quinoa instead of bulgur wheat. Try it using your favorite tabbouleh salad recipe—you might like it even better! (I do.)

⚡ Teriyaki sauce (Read the label, but most contain wheat.)

⚡ Tortillas, flour, whole-wheat, and most "wraps" (Corn tortillas are gluten-free.)

⊘ Triticale, a wheat/rye hybrid grain

U

⊘ Udon, wheat noodles

⊘ Unbleached flour, made from wheat

V

⚡ Veggie bacon (Almost all of them contain wheat gluten.)

⚡ Veggie burgers (Most but not all contain wheat gluten; see Chapter 9 for Eve's vegetarian picks.)

⚡ Veggie "crumbles" or textured vegetable protein designed to resemble ground beef (Many versions contain wheat gluten, although you can find pure soy TVP, including one by Bob's Red Mill.)

⚡ Veggie hot dogs, deli meats, etc. (Many but not all contain wheat gluten. See Chapter 9 for a gluten-free version by Lightlife.)

⚡ Veggie sausages (Most contain wheat gluten, but Chapter 9 lists one gluten-free option by Gardenburger.)

W

⚡ Waffles (Most frozen varieties and waffle mixes contain gluten, but find out more about Van's in Chapter 9.)

🚫 Wheat

🚫 Wheat beer

🚫 Wheat berries

🚫 Wheat bran

🚫 Wheat flour

🚫 Wheat germ

🚫 Wheat germ oil

🚫 Wheat gluten

⚡ Wheat grass, could contain seeds

🚫 Wheat nuts

🚫 Wheat protein

🚫 Wheat starch

🚫 Whole wheat flour

⃠   Wonton wrappers (We use rice paper instead.)

⃠   Wraps (Virtually all mainstream brands are made from wheat flour, including flavored wraps. See Chapter 9 for gluten-free versions.)

Y

▲   Yogurt, flavored (Some flavored varieties contain malt. Plain yogurt is fine.)

▲   Yogurt, frozen (This could be flavored with malt, but might be just fine.)

The Least You Need to Know

◆ The list in this chapter guides you toward many of the foods that usually or always contain gluten, so you can be extra careful about what to avoid.

◆ Always read the label—you might be pleasantly surprised to realize that the food you *thought* had gluten really doesn't!

◆ Don't give up on your snack traditions. Find alternatives from these lists and keep your traditions alive.

Part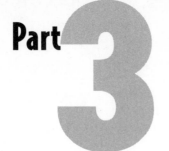

Convenience and Temptation

Do you wonder if you can live without the convenience of processed or packaged foods? In this part, you'll learn all about processed, packaged food (like your favorite frozen dinner or canned soup), and ways to determine whether you can eat it or not. We provide a guide to some of our favorite gluten-free processed and packaged food products. And we're sure you'll discover some new favorites! What about beer and alcohol? Is this a temptation you'll have to give up? Read on .... You'll also get a pep talk here, for those times when gluten-free eating seems too complicated. We can do it, and so can you!

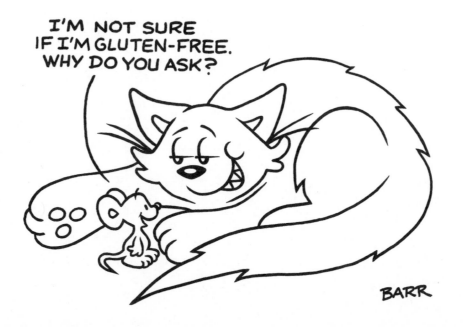

Chapter 8

Processed, Packaged Foods

In This Chapter

- ◆ Twenty-first century Americans love packaged food
- ◆ Refresh your memory about reading the labels on processed, packaged food
- ◆ Processed, packaged foods that probably do or probably don't have gluten

If you didn't mind sticking to plain rice and corn, alternative grains like quinoa and amaranth, fresh unadorned fruits and vegetables, fresh meat, fresh eggs, and fresh milk, eating gluten-free would be pretty simple.

But that's not easy to do in twenty-first century North America. Convenience foods are everywhere, and processed food can be a real conundrum for anybody who needs to eat gluten-free. It's so *easy*. It's so *quick*. And sometimes, you just don't feel like cooking a big dinner. You just want to whip a Lean Cuisine into the microwave or throw some frozen chicken fingers into the oven so the kids stop whining. Been there, done that!

But many (and we mean *many*) of the convenient processed foods you know and might very well love contain gluten. Wheat is an inexpensive source of nutrition, so food manufacturers use it and use it often. In this chapter, we fill you in on some of the things to watch out for when you buy mainstream packaged foods.

Reading the Looooooong Label

Check out your favorite processed food, and you may be surprised at how *long* the list of ingredients is. In Chapter 4, we talked about reading food labels, so let's just touch on some brief reminders about what to remember when scanning those lists on packaged food.

In many cases, wheat will be listed toward the beginning. For example, I'm looking at a product (which will remain anonymous) with an exceptionally long ingredients list that begins like this:

INGREDIENTS: CRUST: Enriched flour (wheat flour, malted barley flour ...)

See, that's all you need to read.

Here's another one, from a product typically sold in the health food section:

INGREDIENTS: Textured vegetable protein (wheat gluten ...).

You can stop now. Even though the list is much longer, you know from this first part that you can't eat the food.

Now let's look at another example, a box of Amy's Kitchen Cheese Enchiladas, a staple in my freezer. On this product, you don't have to read the ingredients list because on the front of the package, it says "No Gluten Ingredients." Although as of this printing, the "gluten-free" (or similar) statement on the front of a package isn't regulated, well-known manufacturers don't just slap it on without thinking. They put that label on food because they don't use gluten ingredients.

And that regulatory situation will change very soon. The FDA is currently developing a ruling that will define the use of the term "gluten-free" on the labels of FDA-regulated packaged food. You can check out the status of that ruling here on the FDA's page called Questions and Answers on the Gluten-Free Labeling Proposed Rule: www.cfsan.fda.gov/~dms/glutqa.html.

We don't currently know what the new rule will contain when it is finally in place, but the fact that the FDA has decided to regulate this term is good news for anyone eating gluten-free. It's an extra level of assurance that when a product says "gluten-free," you know exactly what it means.

Fearless Eater

I try to eat mostly natural, unprocessed food. I really do try. But I also think packaged food is kind of, well … fun! (I blame my mother.) I love getting a snack and then slowly opening up the little package as if it's a present.

So imagine my happy surprise when I found out that some of my favorite packaged foods are gluten-free, including plain tortilla chips, salsa (some brands may have gluten, but my favorites don't), plain rice cakes (I love them with almond butter and orange marmalade), Terra brand vegetable chips, Lärabar brand fruit and nut bars, Cheetos (my kids in particular are very happy that I will still buy these), Amy's Kitchen cheese enchiladas, Nestle hot cocoa mix, salted peanuts, and Nestle Toll House semi-sweet chocolate chips! (Some chocolate chips may have gluten, but thank the chocolate gods, so far these do not.)

But back to those cheese enchiladas. If you decide to read the ingredients list anyway, just to be sure, you'll see:

Cheddar and organic jack cheeses, organic corn tortillas (organic white corn cooked in water with a trace of lime), filtered water, organic onions, organic tomato puree, black olives, organic sweet rice flour, expeller pressed high oleic safflower oil, organic green chiles, spices, organic bell peppers, sea salt, organic garlic. **Contains milk.**

But wait a minute … just below that you will see some more information. It says:

Individuals with Food Allergies: This product is made in a facility that processes foods containing wheat, soy, tree nuts, and seeds. Amy's Kitchen does not use any peanuts, fish, shellfish, or eggs.

Can you still eat the product? I would. It isn't made with gluten-containing ingredients, and from what I know of this company, they would follow good manufacturing practices to prevent cross-contamination. They are committed to providing healthy and safe food, so I trust them. Some people may want to be extra cautious and only eat foods from a dedicated facility, although this can become limiting. Many others don't worry about the issue of cross-contamination from companies they trust. It all depends on how you feel about the issue and what level of risk you are willing to take.

So here's the short version: if you want to eat a particular packaged food, remember the following:

◆ If the product has a "Contains" statement after the ingredients list that says "Contains wheat" (or something to that effect), then no, you don't have to read the label because you know right off that you can't eat it.

◆ If the product does not have a "Contains" statement that reveals wheat, then yes, you do have to read that long ingredients list and look for wheat, barley, rye, malt, or oats (for more on oats, see Chapter 5). Keep reading, all the way to the end!

Remember that because of the Food Allergen Labeling and Consumer Protection Act (FALCPA), as of January 1, 2006, all foods regulated by the FDA containing any of eight common allergens including wheat must clearly state this on the label, so as we've said in other parts of this book, reading the label is a lot easier than it used to be. You don't have to decipher a lot of complicated language. You just have to look for the word "wheat."

And, while FALCPA doesn't address rye, barley, malt, and oats, the law does require manufacturers to list all ingredients on the label. Rye and oats wouldn't normally be listed in any other form than "rye" and "oats" (or something similar like "rye flour" or "rolled oats"). As for malted barley or malt, most of the time, it will be listed as some form of malt on the label.

Yes, that can take some time when the label's long, but it's an unfortunate necessity if you are going to eat processed food. Of course, you can choose *not* to eat processed food, and some people who eat gluten-free make that very choice. But if you are like us (and most gluten-free eaters), at least occasionally, you'll be perusing that label.

Don't Worry, Be Happy

Despite what you may have read in well-meaning but outdated sources, ingredients you may see on a food label of an FDA-regulated product that you really don't have to worry about *unless* wheat is included in the ingredients list or in a separate Contains statement include the following:

◆ MSG (monosodium glutamate)

◆ Citric acid

◆ Mono and diglycerides

◆ Starch (food only)

◆ Distilled alcohol

◆ Distilled vinegar

- Alcohol-based flavorings and extracts

- Dextrose

- Glucose

- Maltose

- Glucose syrup

- Spice

- Dextrin

- Modified food starch

- Coloring

Read the Label

In a USDA-regulated food (meat, poultry, or egg products), dextrin, modified food starch, caramel color, and glucose syrup could rarely be derived from wheat and caramel color could potentially be derived from barley malt. Also, in FDA-regulated food products, natural flavoring and caramel color could potentially be derived from barley malt.

Packaged Food Round-Up

It would be nice if we could make a list for you of every single processed food out there by name and tell you exactly which ones do and do not contain gluten. Unfortunately, that's impossible because manufacturers change their formulas often, so a product that contains gluten one day might not contain it the next, and vice versa.

What we can do, however, is give you a list of the *kinds* of packaged foods that *usually* contain gluten, and the *kinds* of packaged foods that *usually don't* contain gluten.

Remember, however, that the label on the actual product you plan to eat is the ultimate authority. *You must read the label before eating the food.*

As long as we can all agree on that, then here is a list to help guide you in your search for the perfect gluten-free convenience food. It certainly isn't inclusive—you probably can think of more things to add—but this is a general roundup of the common packaged food familiar to many people.

You'll notice some crossover in this list because some foods fall into several categories. This list only covers packaged food. For more comprehensive lists covering a wider range of foods, check out Chapters 6 and 7. For lists of gluten-free foods, see Chapter 9.

Frozen Foods That *Probably* Contain Gluten

Frozen bread, rolls, or other premade baked goods

Frozen breaded anything

Frozen breakfast breads of all types

Frozen chicken nuggets

Frozen chicken patties

Frozen chicken-fried anything

Frozen dinners

Frozen family-style meals, like pans of lasagna, enchiladas, macaroni and cheese, etc.

Frozen fish sticks and fish pieces

Frozen gravy packets

Frozen meat balls

Frozen pancakes

Frozen skillet meals

Frozen vegetables in sauce (some are just fine—read labels)

Frozen waffles

Frozen whole turkey injected with basting solution

Vegetarian breakfast "meats"

Veggie burgers

Frozen Foods That *Probably Don't* Contain Gluten

Frozen chicken breasts or chicken pieces, plain (not breaded, seasoned, or in a sauce)

Frozen fish, unbreaded and unseasoned

Good for You _____

Try making fish sticks or chicken fingers by cutting fresh fish or chicken filets into strips, then dipping them into egg whites and rolling them in cornmeal mixed with sesame seeds and a little chili powder. Bake until crispy. It's almost as quick as opening a package.

Frozen shrimp, plain

Frozen vegetables, plain, unseasoned

Frozen whole poultry _not_ injected with basting solution

Ice cream without gluten-containing ingredients or malt flavoring

Canned, Jarred, and Bottled Foods That *Probably* Contain Gluten

Boston brown bread

Canned soup (some canned soups are fine—read labels)

Chili

Cream sauces, like Alfredo, hollandaise, etc.

Dinners, like canned ravioli, corned beef hash, etc.

Gravy

Meat in sauce or gravy

Shoyu sauce

Soy sauce

Vegetables in sauce (some are just fine—read labels)

Canned and Jarred Foods That *Probably Don't* Contain Gluten

Applesauce, natural

Beans, water-packed

Canned tomatoes

Canned tuna, water- or oil-packed

Canned vegetables, water-packed

Fish sauce (read labels carefully)

Fruit, water-packed

Jarred vegetables, water-packed

Pickled vegetables

Pickles

Sauerkraut

Fearless Eater

One of my favorite health-food manufacturers is Amy's Kitchen because their food tastes so good! Lots of it has gluten, but lots of it doesn't, too, and their website makes it very easy to search for the gluten-free products Amy's makes. Visit here: www.amyskitchen.com/products/special_diets.php, and click on "Gluten-Free." You'll also see their gluten-free symbol on all the product listings on the website, making it even easier to spot the foods you can eat. Enjoy! (And don't miss the Organic Medium Chili with Vegetables. Delicious!)

Packaged Dry Goods That *Probably* Contain Gluten

Bagels

Bakery items

Baking mix

Bread

Bread crumbs

Bread sticks

Brownie mix

Cake mix

Chili mix

Coffee cake

Cookie mix

Croutons

Dinner rolls

Doughnuts

English muffins

Flour tortillas

Pancake mix

Pasta

Pasta mixes

Pastry

Pie crust

Ramen noodles

Scones

Stuffing mix

Sweet rolls

Waffle mix

Wraps

Fearless Eater
We were on the road, cross-country, and I was hungry. We stopped at a gas station somewhere in the middle of Illinois, and I wandered around, looking for something I could eat. I passed the doughnuts, of course, the snack cakes, and cereal bars. Then I started reading labels. Ben said, "We have to get going." I said, "Just a minute! This is research!" I actually found a lot of things to feed the need: plain beef jerky (the teriyaki flavor had wheat), potato chips, caramel corn, cashews, three flavors of corn chips, a package of mini rice cakes, and a Diet Coke. Ben said, "You know, just because it doesn't have gluten doesn't mean you have to buy it." I said, "But I'm hungry. And did I mention this is research?" So I bought it all, and we were happily fed for the rest of the trip.

Packaged Dry Goods That *Probably Don't* Contain Gluten

Corn tortillas

Rice, plain

Rice cakes (some contain gluten so check labels carefully)

Rice noodles

Taco shells, made from corn

Snack Foods That *Probably* Contain Gluten

Cereal bars

Cookies

Crackers

Cupcakes

Dried dates, could be dusted with gluten-containing oat flour

Energy bars (some are just fine—read the label)

Granola bars

Pretzels

Snack cakes

Toaster pastries

Good for You

Many food manufacturers are very helpful about which foods they make do and don't contain gluten. In fact, many print lists on their websites, updated regularly, regarding which foods are gluten-free. One my kids encourage me to check often is the FritoLay site's "Products Not Containing Gluten" page. Find it here: www. fritolay.com/fl/flstore/cgi-bin/dietary_choices.htm and click on "Products Not Containing Gluten."

Snack Foods That *Probably Don't* Contain Gluten

Beef jerky, original flavor (Some of the flavored varieties contain soy sauce with wheat.)

Dried fruit (except dates)

Fruit snacks

Nuts, plain

Popcorn

Potato chips, plain

Rice crackers

Sunflower seeds

Tortilla chips, plain

Vegetable chips

Beverages That *Probably* Contain Gluten

Beer

Malted milk

Fearless Eater

I'm often reading in other books and on the Internet how all these flavored coffees and flavored beverages contain gluten. Actually, in my experience, most beverages *probably don't* contain gluten, other than malted milk and beer. In my own cabinets and refrigerator, right this moment, none of the following contain any gluten: instant flavored coffee, instant chai, flavored tea, hot cocoa mix, several varieties of diet and nondiet soda, canned lemonade, and canned flavored iced tea. Now, don't get me wrong—some of these had some weird ingredients and long lists. One of the sodas contained glycerol ester of wood rosin and brominated vegetable oil. Huh? I'm not sure I want to drink *that* anymore. But no gluten.

Of course, manufacturers can change their recipes at any time, and maybe the next time I buy instant flavored coffee or canned iced tea, it will suddenly have gluten (and you, of course, should read your own labels every time). But so far, so good!

Beverages That *Probably Don't* Contain Gluten

Coffee, plain

Tea, plain, black, green, white, etc.

Soft drinks

Sports drinks

The natural next step after talking about processed foods with and without gluten is to take a good look at the huge proliferation of packaged foods that are now being manufactured specifically to be gluten-free. For more on this fascinating new world of gluten-free convenience, continue on to Chapter 9.

The Least You Need to Know

◆ It's hard to avoid processed food.

◆ Many processed and packaged foods contain gluten.

◆ If you know what to look for, you can find convenient processed, packaged food that doesn't have gluten.

A Quick Guide to Gluten-Free Packaged Food

In This Chapter

◆ All that stuff you miss

◆ Understanding the nature of gluten-free foods

◆ Eve's Favorites

◆ Tricia's Favorites

What was the first food *you* missed when you went gluten-free? Or if you haven't begun yet, what do you think you will miss most? For me, it was bread … and toast. Then it was cookies. And when I went to a party and couldn't eat the yummy-looking birthday cake, that was my next fond nostalgic longing. But then … I discovered gluten-free packaged food.

Sure, you can get by just fine eating nothing but fruits, vegetables, rice, corn, fresh meat, and plain dairy products. You can cook everything at home, and you'd probably be very healthy. But sometimes, you just really want a brownie. Or a big stack of pancakes. Or a really good pizza crust.

So here come gluten-free products to the rescue! In this chapter, we present some of the delicious and excellent gluten-free products available to you and also give you short lists of some of our personal favorites.

Gluten-Free Products: The Pros and Cons

I admit that when I first discovered the gluten-free section in my grocery store, I went a little crazy. "Cookies! Cake mixes! Bread! Pancakes! I need to try them all! It's a *business expense!*"

But then I got to the checkout counter and saw the total on the cash register. Business expense or not, I still had to pay the bill, and gluten-free food can be expensive. In fact, most of the time, the gluten-free equivalent of a "regular" food (like a loaf of bread, a package of cake mix, or a box of cookies) will cost more than the gluten-filled version. This is a specialty market, and it costs more to get quality ingredients and make these products, so it only makes sense. Nobody is trying to rip you off; it's just the nature of the specialty food market.

Good for You _____

Can you write off gluten-free foods as a medical expense? Consult your tax accountant to be sure, but you might be able to write off the difference in price between certain gluten-free products, like bread and cereal, and the regular versions of these products if you have an official diagnosis of celiac disease from your doctor. We can't give you financial advice, but come tax time, it certainly doesn't hurt to ask. You can also check out the IRS information publication regarding medical expenses here: www.irs.gov/taxtopics/tc502.html.

The good part of the equation is that if you want to be budget-conscious, you can center your diet around healthy home-cooked foods and just indulge in the gluten-free packaged foods on occasion … you know, when you *really* need that cookie.

Also, the first time you taste gluten-free baked goods, you may not like them very much because you will be comparing them to the foods you ate in the past. Remember that foods made from rice flour, corn flour, arrowroot, potato starch, and other gluten-free grains, like quinoa and buckwheat, can't possibly taste the same as foods made from wheat flour because they aren't made from wheat flour.

The trick to appreciating and enjoying gluten-free foods is to taste them on their own terms. The more you try and taste and become accustomed to the flavors characteristic of alternative grains, the more you will develop your gluten-free palate and appreciate these foods for what they are. So be patient and keep tasting. You'll soon find your favorites. (We did!)

Gluten-Free Packaged Food List

What products can you find that are gluten-free? Plenty! We've found these items in our own grocery or natural foods stores or online, completely gluten-free and conveniently packaged for your eating pleasure:

- Bagels
- Barbeque sauce
- Bouillon cubes
- Bread
- Bread mix
- Bread sticks
- Breakfast bars
- Brownie mix
- Brownies
- Cake mix
- Candy
- Chocolate chips
- Cold cereal
- Communion wafers
- Cookies
- Crackers (lots of flavors)
- Crisp bread (like rye crisps, without the rye)
- Croutons

- Curry sauce
- Energy bars
- Flavored rice mixes
- Rice (or other non-gluten-grain) flour tortillas
- Frozen dinners
- Gravy mix
- Hot cereal
- Instant noodle bowls
- Lasagna
- Macaroni and cheese mix (in the box, just like you're used to)
- Muffins
- Mustard—lots of flavors
- Nutritional supplements (like vitamin/mineral formulas)
- Oatmeal (most commercial varieties in the United States are contaminated with gluten, but you can buy gluten-free varieties)
- Pancake mix
- Pasta dinners
- Pasta/noodles
- Pizza
- Pretzels
- Scones
- Snack chips
- Soup
- Soy sauce
- Spaghetti
- Steak sauce
- Sundae topping

- Sweet & sour sauce

- Thai peanut sauce

- Trail mix

- Veggie burgers

- Veggie hot dogs

- Waffle cones

- Waffle mix

Where to Find Gluten-Free Products

And where do you find all these wonderful gluten-free versions of your favorite foods? That used to be tricky, but regular grocery stores seem to be continually expanding their gluten-free sections, so depending on where you live, you may be able to find plenty of gluten-free products where you normally shop. If not, many health food stores and food co-ops stock lots of good gluten-free food.

Whole Foods and Trader Joe's, two major health food chain stores in many states, now both carry a wide variety of gluten-free products, and continue to expand their selections. And of course, you can always order gluten-free food online. Appendix B lists lots of gluten-free food manufacturers, or browse these websites, which sell many different gluten-free products:

- The Gluten-Free Mall: This website offers a wide variety of gluten-free products from many different manufacturers, which can be ordered from this website. Look here: www.glutenfreemall.com.

- Shop Gluten Free: This website also lists a wide variety of gluten-free products from many different manufacturers. Browse here: www.shopglutenfree.com.

You can also browse around the Whole Foods Market Gluten-free Bakehouse here: www.wholefoodsmarket.com/products/bakery/gf_bakehouse.html.

Eve's Picks for the Best-Tasting Gluten-Free Packaged Foods

I admit it: I love to eat, and I love to try new food, too. As much as I try to eat all-natural, home-cooked food, just something about packaged food feels somehow fun to me … like opening a present. So did I balk for one second at the chance to try tons of gluten-free packaged foods? You better believe I didn't! Of course, it was all for you. Well, okay, it was also for me.

To be honest, I didn't find every gluten-free product I tried delicious. But many were excellent! I know there are many, many other delicious gluten-free products I haven't tried yet, but this is my list of favorites so far—the gluten-free products I'll continue to buy.

Also, please be aware that everybody's taste buds are different. First of all, you may not be used to the taste of foods made without wheat yet, and it may take some time to get used to them and start to like them. That happens to almost everyone. But even beyond that point, you might not agree with Tricia or me about some of the brands we love. Of course, that's perfectly fine! Tricia and I don't always like the same brands, either. We each have our tastes, and you have yours. In the next few sections, we list the gluten-free foods we enjoy. You may enjoy them, too, or you may prefer others. The point is to keep trying things until you find the ones that satisfy *you*.

> **Fearless Eater**
>
> When I first tasted gluten-free bread, I didn't like it *at all*. It was crumbly and spongy. Yuck. (I won't mention any names.) But then I tried a few other brands and began to get used to the texture, and now I don't mind it at all, toasted with peanut butter or cheese on top. However, even better than the prebaked stuff is the bread you can make from bread mixes. Although brands vary, some are fluffy, soft, and delicious, especially warm from the oven with butter or toasted with jam. It's how I always eat bread now—it's worth the extra time to bake it. I particularly recommend Pamela's wheat-free bread mix. It makes great bread but also pizza crust and pie crust. Just follow the instructions on the box. I also recommend Bob's Red Mill Homemade Wonderful Gluten-Free Bread Mix. It's really delicious, too.

Glutino, Kinnikinnick, and Ener-G

These gluten-free food manufacturers aren't the only ones, or the only good ones, but they are three of my favorites. Glutino makes some delicious products that replace many of the things I missed. I especially like Glutino's pretzels—I don't even like pretzels that much, but I think the Glutino pretzels are tastier than the regular kind. I also love their sesame bread sticks (plenty of crunch), the gluten-free rusks (a great substitute for crackers or rye crisp), their honey-nut cereal (perfect for late-night sweet cravings without all the calories), and their cookies. They also make croutons, for those of you who really miss that bready crunch in your salad. Glutino is in Quebec, and all the packages have French on one side and English on the other, so you'll feel *so* sophisticated eating those lemon wafers and vanilla dream bites (or *Bouchées Caprice à la Vanille*, as I like to call them!). Find out more at www.glutino.com.

As for Kinnikinnick, a few weeks ago when I looked into the frozen-foods part of the health food section of my grocery store and saw gluten-free donuts, I thought I'd died and gone to heaven. I bought a package of the vanilla dipped and the chocolate dipped, went home, brewed some coffee, and warmed one donut of each flavor in the microwave. Ahh … that was a good day!

I also think their brown sandwich bread is terrific and just the ticket when I don't have time to bake bread. Everything Kinnikinnick makes is gluten-free, so you always know you're safe with their foods. They make everything in a dedicated gluten-free facility. Find out more about them at www.kinnikinnick.com.

Ener-G makes lots of different products for restricted diets, including delicious pre-baked gluten-free foods like donuts, dinner rolls, cookies, and brownies, as well as baking mixes and baking ingredients. I really enjoyed a pan of their super-chocolately brownies. No, I didn't eat the whole pan myself. (Just half.) Find out more here: www.ener-g.com.

Amy's Kitchen and Ian's

Amy's Kitchen doesn't make exclusively gluten-free products—a lot of their products contain wheat and all are vegetarian. But if you love the convenience of frozen dinners, you'll go crazy for this company's products, especially if you aren't a big meat eater. I believe I've mentioned several times how much I enjoy the cheese enchiladas, but I also like the Indian Mattar Panner (I just finished a tray for my lunch while writing this—it has just the right amount of spicy), and the rice-crust pizza. I'm also *all* about the medium chili with vegetables—a totally delicious gluten-free favorite in my house. Dip your corn chips in it!

Amy's also has a search feature on their website that allows you to search specifically for gluten-free foods. As of today, according to the website, they have 60 gluten-free products. Look here to find them: www.amys.com/special_diets/celiac.php. Scroll down to the "Amy's Kitchen Products" section, and click on "Gluten-Free Products."

When it comes to kid food, Ian's is great. Not all their products are gluten-free but they make delicious gluten-free fish sticks, fries, sweet potato fries, chicken nuggets, and popcorn turkey corn dogs. My kids loved these. They even have a gluten-free version of those "kid meals" in trays that kids think are so fun. Find out more about them at www.iansnaturalfoods.com.

Good Baking Mixes

One of the best gluten-free baking mixes out there (and one of the most popular) is Pamela's amazing pancake mix. Not only do my kids love it, but they also love it *better than* regular pancake mix or even the from-scratch pancakes I used to make back in the gluten days. I sprinkle a few chocolate chips over each pancake (are you sensing a theme here?), and they go crazy for them.

Also tops on my list are Pamela's chocolate cake mix, chocolate brownie mix, and the fantastic bread mix, that makes soft, delicious, bready bread and really good pizza crust, too. Find them at www.pamelasproducts.com.

Bob's Red Mill makes a lot of baking mixes, and they aren't all gluten-free, but their bread mix is fantastic. They also have delicious cornbread mix, cinnamon raisin bread mix, chocolate cake mix, biscuit mixes, and chocolate chip cookie mix. If you feel like baking, consult Bob. Find more information about their gluten-free products here: www.bobsredmill.com/gluten_free_info.php.

Snack Stuff

Can I tell you how much I love Pamela for making the most delicious gluten-free cookies? I particularly love the chocolate chip mini cookies, the ginger snap mini cookies, the peanut butter cookies, and the chocolate chocolate chunk cookies. These are just the ticket when I just *really* need something sweet and comforting. In the car today, my youngest polished off the rest of the bag of chocolate chip mini cookies. You see, I'm finally learning to pack a bag of gluten-free snacks before we hit the road, and let me just tell you that my bag is brimming with Pamela's products.

Speaking of snacking away from home, I first discovered Lärabars in my local coffee shop. Every week after yoga class my friend Rachel and I go there, and we used to get croissants or cinnamon rolls with our coffee. Since I went gluten-free, however, I *have watched Rachel eat cinnamon rolls*. That is, until I noticed the box of Lärabars next to the cash register. "These probably aren't gluten-free," I muttered, picking one up, somewhat resignedly, to read the label. And what did I see? Lo and behold, the label said gluten-free! It also said the bars were organic, raw, nondairy, and free of all kinds of other stuff, so I thought, hmmm, how good can this be? It turns out it was *delicious!* A yummy, gooey, nutrient-dense bar of dates and nuts, this really satisfies. In fact, they even had *cinnamon roll flavor*, so now Rachel and I each enjoy a cinnamon roll with our coffee again, or, at least, we each enjoy our own versions.

Other Lärabar flavors I particular like include the apple pie, pecan pie, cherry pie, pistachio, cashew cookie, banana, ginger snap, lemon, and chocolate mole, which has cinnamon and chili peppers! It's unusual, but delicious!

Lärabar also has a yummy line of bars called jŏcalat. These are made from dates, nuts, and organic cocoa, in great flavors: chocolate orange, chocolate coffee, chocolate mint, and of course, just plain chocolate. They are so healthy that they will make you feel great about fulfilling your chocolate craving. (At least, I feel pretty virtuous.)

Health Valley makes many delicious, healthy foods, but many of them have gluten. However, the Rice Bran crackers are gluten-free, and I love them with peanut butter or almond butter. They stand in very well for graham crackers, in my opinion.

Pasta and Pizza

I love pasta and really missed spaghetti until I tried Lundberg Family Farms organic brown rice pasta. Even my kids liked it. It isn't the precise texture of semolina spaghetti but it's darn close. I had it last night with olive oil, salt, and pepper and felt very satisfied. Lundberg Family Farms makes many other delicious gluten-free products, including rice mixes and rice cakes, risottos in many flavors, rice chips, hot rice cereal, rice milk, and several shapes of rice pasta. Check out the list here: www.lundberg.com/info/glutenfree.shtml.

Another of my favorites is Thai Kitchen. You won't miss ramen noodles with Thai Kitchen's rice noodle bowls. I like the mushroom flavor. Add in your own fresh veggies for an even heartier lunch. Some of Thai Kitchen's other boxed dinners are also gluten-free, like the Thai Peanut meal kit and the Pad Thai meal kit. All their rice mixes are also gluten-free. Find out exactly what's what on their allergy information page on the website. Go here: www.thaikitchen.com/allergyinfo.html.

Good for You _____

For those who really miss their oatmeal—because hot rice cereal, although delicious, just isn't the same—you can buy oats that are pure and uncontaminated by wheat, rye, or barley. Neither Tricia nor I have tried these, but you might want to check them out. Find them at www.glutenfreeoats.com and at www.pureoats.com.

As for pizza, Van Harden makes a pizza with a crust made from cheese. It's a thin crust pizza, and mighty tasty, in my opinion. They have cheese, pepperoni, and sausage flavors, made right here in Iowa but available in Hy-Vee stores in seven Midwestern states (if your Hy-Vee store doesn't have it, ask them and they can order it), or online through www.vanharden.com (although the shipping charges are steep).

Lou Malnati's makes a crustless pizza with a sausage base available at 25 pizzerias in the Chicago area, or available online at www.tastesofchicago.com/product/392/4. I haven't tried it, but sausage lovers might find it just the thing.

Or try Amy's Kitchen rice crust cheese pizza, which is widely available. I think it tastes nice.

Gluten-Free Vegetarian

I eat mostly vegetarian so I was crushed to learn most veggie burgers, veggie sausages, and veggie "crumbles" contain gluten—it gives these products that chewy, meatlike texture. However, after a little hunting, I found a few great vegetarian products without gluten, so of course I'll share my finds with you.

- Wildwood Organics Tofu Veggie Burgers are delicious and gluten-free. These are my favorites. Find them here: www.wildwoodfoods.com.

- I also enjoy Sunshine Burgers: www.sunshineburger.com.

- Gardenburger now has a veggie burger without gluten: the Black Bean Chipotle Veggie Pattie. As of press time, their website claims the Flame-Grilled Burgers are also gluten-free, but the ingredients list includes malt extract, which *does contain gluten*, so avoid this variety. They also make a gluten-free Veggie Breakfast Sausage, so you can have sausage and eggs again, without the meat *or* the gluten! Find out more at www.gardenburger.com.

- Amy's Kitchen makes a Bistro Burger that is both gluten-free and dairy-free. I couldn't find it in my store but you might be able to find it in yours. Not all Amy's veggie burgers are gluten-free, however, so be sure to find the Bistro Burger specifically. Go to www.amyskitchen.com.

◆ If you just want a hot dog but you don't eat meat, try Lightlife tofu pups. They are one of the few gluten-free versions of vegetarian hot dogs. Lightlife also makes a gluten-free organic tempeh, which is a great protein source for vegetarians. Find out more at www.lightlife.com.

Tricia's Picks for the Best-Tasting Gluten-Free Packaged Foods

Tricia has been eating gluten-free for many more years than I have (in fact, my gluten-free adventure is better counted in months rather than years), so it's only natural that she has her favorites, too. After reading about them, I'm ready to expand my gluten-free horizons even further! I bet you will be, too.

Enjoy Life Foods and Tinkyada Brown Rice Pasta

Tricia loves anything by Enjoy Life Foods. They make ready-made bagels, granola, snack bars, cookies, and trail mix. Tricia is especially fond of the chocolate chip cookies and calls them her "absolute favorite gluten-free snack food." In fact, Tricia's son Marcus (who does not follow a gluten-free diet) loves these cookies as well.

Enjoy Life also enriches their bagels, granola, and snack bars with a variety of vitamins and minerals for extra nutrition. Those yummy snacks seem like downright virtuous choices! All products manufactured by this company are gluten-free and produced in a gluten-free facility. Their website is www.enjoylifefoods.com.

Tricia also says Tinkyada brown rice pasta isn't mushy and holds up well in baked pasta dishes, too. I tried it, and she's right! It's readily available in natural foods stores, and in fact, it has become my gluten-free pasta brand of choice, too. Their website is www.tinkyada.com.

Good for You _____

What's a Catholic with celiac disease supposed to do come communion time? Under Canon law, communion wafers must contain wheat. One brand has been specially formulated to comply with Canon law but also contains very low levels of gluten. Find them at http://benedictinesisters.org, then click on "low gluten altar bread."

Quinoa in Any Form ... Any Brand

This naturally gluten-free "grain" is a nutritional powerhouse and is delicious, too. It's incredibly easy to make and versatile because it takes on the flavor of whatever you cook with it. However, Tricia suggests starting out your quinoa adventure by thinking of it as a replacement for rice. It works well playing the same role in a meal—you can make it into a pilaf or eat it with a stir-fry, for example. Tricia suggests cooking up a batch with a gluten-free chicken stock instead of water for extra flavor and trying it out. Experiment, then look for products (like pasta) that use quinoa. Quinoa is readily available in grocery and natural foods stores.

Breakfast!

Tricia loves Van's brand waffles and uses them for sandwiches, too. Made with whole-grain brown rice flour, these waffles are nutrient-packed, too (you know nutritionists, always looking for that nutritious food!). Van's also makes gluten-containing waffles, so be extra careful which one you grab, but their gluten-free varieties are clearly marked "gluten-free" and are available in natural foods stores as well as some grocery stores. Their website is www.vansintl.com.

If you love chocolate and you haven't tried Genisoy's peanut butter fudge bars yet, then what are you waiting for? Tricia eats one of these bars, which are fortified with a wide variety of vitamins and minerals, every day. Only two of the Genisoy variety bars are currently gluten-free: the peanut butter fudge bar and the creamy peanut yogurt bar. They aren't specifically advertised as gluten-free, but if you look at the ingredients list, you will see that they don't contain any gluten ingredients. Their line of protein crunch bars are also gluten-free, but read the ingredients list each time to be sure. Their website is www.genisoy.com.

Finding Your Own Favorites

We hope we've been able to guide you toward some of the foods we like, but you may not always agree with our tastes, and you may find other products we haven't mentioned that you love. The best way to get started is to just start tasting.

We've also listed names and websites for gluten-free food manufacturers in Appendix B. That's a great place to go next. Good luck, and happy tasting!

The Least You Need to Know

◆ Practically all the baked goods and other foods you can't eat anymore are available in gluten-free versions at stores near you or online from specialty gluten-free manufacturers.

◆ Because gluten-free foods often taste different than their gluten-filled counterparts, you have to get used to a different taste, and you'll enjoy them more if you take them on their own terms and don't compare them.

◆ Try different brands to find your favorites, and check out Appendix B for good resources.

10

Gluten-Free Beer and Alcohol

In This Chapter

◆ Beer is back!

◆ Other gluten-free alcoholic beverages

◆ A cautionary tale about cocktails

You teetotalers can skip this chapter because we're going to talk about alcohol: beer, wine, liquor, and cocktails. If you avoid the stuff entirely, then this chapter isn't for you, but if you enjoy your happy hour, your after-work cocktail, your weekend football beer, your wine with dinner, or that relaxing nightcap, this chapter is just for you.

You've probably already heard the nasty rumors … that people who eat gluten-free *can't drink beer.* (Gasp!) Is it so? Can't I please tell you it isn't so? Well, sort of … it used to be true, until a few forward-thinking brewers entered the gluten-free market. So let's start with beer because we know you're worried. You want to *know:* is football season over for good?

Gluten-Free Beer: Hope for the Thirsty

It's so crisp. So refreshing. So *necessary* while mowing the lawn. Do you really have to give up beer if you have to give up gluten?

Traditionally (and I mean for thousands of years), beer has been made out of grain—usually barley. Barley is just right for brewing beer because it has a lot of natural sugars the yeast can convert to alcohol and very few proteins to clog up the brew. But it does have gluten. But barley isn't the only brewable grain. In Africa, for example, people have traditionally brewed beer from sorghum—and sorghum is gluten-free. So is rice, and corn, and millet—all potential sources of beer.

One of the things that seems to upset a lot of people the most when they first learn they must eat a gluten-free diet is that they can't drink beer. And I'm one of them! I wrote a book on craft beer appreciation, and I love beer—light, crisp, wheat beers, deep chocolately stouts, girly fruit beers, manly Imperial IPAs, bitter or sweet, light or dark, I love to taste them, evaluate them, and rate them.

No beer? Frankly, I almost didn't agree to do this book for this single reason. But then I found out a secret: a few brewers have been working away to produce some delicious gluten-free beers, made from other grain sources that don't have gluten: sorghum, rice, and buckwheat. Hallelujah! I can taste and evaluate beer again!

Fearless Eater

To be quite frank, I'm not much of a football fan, but this year, when the Bears played the Colts, I had to get excited—Iowa is all about the Bears (since we don't have our own football team), and Ben is from Indiana, which is die-hard Colts country, so obviously, we had to have a party. But what was I supposed to drink? Ah-ha ... Anheuser Busch to the rescue! I drank Redbridge sorghum beer, munched on tortilla chips and salsa, and blended in perfectly with the rest of the crowd. I felt so ... so ... *normal!* Go Bears! (Yes, I know, the Colts won. Ben is still smirking.)

The other good news is that more and more brewers are becoming aware of this growing market of beer lovers who can't stomach barley, so expect more gluten-free beers on the market soon. In this chapter, I evaluate the gluten-free beers I've tried, so you can find your *new* personal favorite.

Now, before you jump right in, I want to warn you that gluten-free beer doesn't taste exactly like beer brewed from malted barley. It has a different aftertaste. The trick is not to compare them (although I offer some comparisons in my reviews just to steer you toward the ones you might like). The trick is to judge them entirely on their own, in the spectrum of beers you can now enjoy. Each of the beers I evaluated had interesting, complex flavors, and I really enjoyed them, in their own right. I'm sure you will, too.

Anheuser-Busch Redbridge

Anheuser-Busch knows when a market is growing, and they've recently gotten into the gluten-free market with a sorghum-based beer called Redbridge—the gluten-free beer you're probably most likely to be able to find. This beer pours a deep rich gold color with a nice head. It has a pretty light aroma—doesn't smell like much, but the taste is surprisingly hoppy and rich, with a rich cut-grassy hoppiness, pleasantly bitter.

Redbridge has a quick finish but more taste than I expected … in fact, more taste than some of Anheuser-Busch's more mainstream beers, in my opinion. The nice bitter hoppiness holds up nicely to spicy food. If you like hoppy beers or you used to drink Sam Adams, you might like Redbridge.

Find out more about Redbridge at www.redbridgebeer.com.

Bard's Tale Dragon's Gold

Dragon's Gold claims to be the world's first 100 percent sorghum malt craft-brewed beer. I was able to find this beer in my supermarket in Iowa, and according to the Bard's Tale website, this gluten-free sorghum beer is available in many states across the country from the east coast to the west coast and also internationally.

I think Dragon's Gold has a British-style ale-like taste to it even though it is advertised as a lager. It has a pleasant malty aroma with some floral hoppiness and pours a medium-gold color. The taste is sweet and round, malty with a subtle hop flavor on the finish. I get toffee notes, honey, a hint of butterscotch, and plenty of sparkle—it's definitely sweet and would appeal to someone who likes a maltier beer. I would compare it to Bass or even Boddingtons Pub Ale, but the sorghum definitely gives it a different taste than barley-based beer.

Find out more at www.bardsbeer.com.

Lakefront's New Grist

Lakefront Brewery in Milwaukee recently introduced New Grist, a gluten-free beer brewed from sorghum and rice extract with guaranteed gluten-free yeast grown on molasses. Every batch is tested for gluten prior to fermentation. New Grist pours a brilliant gold. It has a light floral aroma and a crisp, bright flavor with a pleasant grassiness. This is subtle and wispy on the tongue with a hint of lime. If you like Corona with a lime, you'll like New Grist. Drink it on the beach or while mowing the lawn. It's very refreshing.

Check them out at www.newgrist.com.

Nouvelle France's La Messagère

This Canadian import is advertised as a pale-ale-style beer, but this rice and buckwheat beer *sans gluten* is less hoppy than a typical pale ale—lighter and fruitier. La Messagère pours a pale, straw-gold with a dainty head. The rice gives this beer a much lighter and more delicate look and taste than the other gluten-free beers I tried, except perhaps for New Grist.

The aroma is citrusy, mostly lemon with a hint of grapefruit and some subtle floral notes. The beer tastes smooth and tangy, almost like a restrained version of a Flemish ale—it's unusual, so if you like beer with complexity, you'll probably prefer this to some of the American-made gluten-free beers. If you miss citrusy, fruity beers and wheat beers like Blue Moon, you'll probably enjoy La Messagère. You won't need to add a lemon slice, but a slice of orange might be interesting. I tasted this in March, but this would be a great summer, hot-weather beer to drink by the pool.

Check out their website at www.lesbieresnouvellefrance.com.

Sprecher Shakporo

This fire-brewed African-style sorghum and millet ale tastes like a tangy wheat beer with a sharp, puckery, satisfyingly thirst-quenching taste. Shakporo has a citrusy-hoppy aroma and notes of grapefruit, orange peel, fresh grass, and yeast. For people who like beer with a stronger flavor, especially those who used to enjoy wheat beer, sour ales, or funky Belgian beers, this might just make you very happy. It made me very happy. Find out more at www.sprecherbrewery.com.

Belgian Beer from Green's

Since writing a craft beer book, I've been a huge fan of Belgian beer, so I was so excited to hear that Green's brewery, a gluten-free brewery in the UK, was coming out with three gluten-free beers brewed for them in Belgium: a dubbel called Endeavor, a tripel called Quest, and an amber called Discovery. I got samples just in time to get them into the book. Here's the verdict:

First, Discovery, the amber. This all-natural amber beer is made from a millet, rice, buckwheat, and sorghum mixture. It pours a true amber with a light malty aroma. The taste is tangy and sweet, with hints of maple syrup, cola, and ginger. Lots of carbonation, this is very refreshing and tasty. It's 6% alcohol.

Next, Endeavor, the dubbel. Belgian beer fans know dubbels are supposed to be dark and rich. This one pours a deep maple syrup color and although the aroma is light, this one has even more maple flavor than the amber. This is lighter in flavor than a lot of dubbels I've had, but would probably appeal to those who don't like a heavy beer. It has a nice foamy head, hints of black pepper and clove, and a quick finish. It weighs in at 7% alcohol.

Finally, Quest, the tripel. This is usually my favorite style of Belgian beer, and it's my favorite of these three, as well. It pours a bright light gold with lots of bubbles and foam. The aroma is light floral with bread notes, and the taste is crisp and citrusy with a long tangy finish. The yeast flavor is slighter than in some tripels but this is really easy to drink. Watch out, though. The 8.5% alcohol might sneak up on you.

All three of these beers are just recently out and available in many states. For more information on the Green's products available in the United States, see www.merchantduvin.com, and click on "Green's."

Other Gluten-Free Beers

Some other breweries also make gluten-free beers, but I haven't tried them. These include:

◆ Rampano Valley Brewery in New York: rampanovalleybrewery.com. This brewer makes several styles but only one is gluten-free: the award-winning Passover Honey Beer.

◆ O'Brien's Premium Lager: www.obrienbrewing.com.au. This comes from Australia but may be available in the United States at some point soon.

There are more gluten-free beers that are mostly available in other countries, not in the United States, so I haven't listed them here. However, if you really want to get into gluten-free beer, especially while traveling, check out the Gluten Free Beer Festival website: www.glutenfreebeerfestival.com. They review gluten-free beers from all over the world, with lots of great beer-related resources for people who can't drink gluten! Expect more brewers to experiment with gluten-free beer in the future, too—all signs point to gluten-free beer as a big growth market. This list can only get longer.

Hard Cider

Hard cider by definition is wine made primarily from apples or apple concentrate and water. All true hard ciders should be gluten-free. This yummy fermented beverage *looks* like beer and *tastes* like fruit. I enjoy Sutliff Hard Cider, made right here in Iowa, but many other companies make excellent hard ciders, too. Flavored ciders and other malt-based beverages, such as wine coolers and hard lemonade, often contain malt. If you are unsure whether a particular flavored hard cider is gluten-free, contact the manufacturer.

Wine Is Fine

You wine drinkers out there can sit back and relax. Yep, breathe a big sigh of relief: wine is just fine. It doesn't contain gluten and never did.

Wine is not only gluten-free, but probably heart-healthy in moderation (one 4-ounce glass for women or two 4-ounce glasses for men per day), at least according to some studies. Wine also can be a delicious part of gluten-free cooking, adding complex flavor to your favorite savory recipes.

Better yet, most cheese is gluten-free, too! Skip the bread, grab some gluten-free rice crackers and some stinky French cheese, and have a wine tasting. And a lovely evening. Cheers! (By the way, champagne is just fine, too.)

Liquor Is Quicker

As I've mentioned previously, I love beer, but I'm also a big fan of the cocktail—gin martinis, Manhattans, and bourbon highballs are my favorites, but I think it's fun to try new ones (or old ones) whenever I get the chance (in moderation, of course). So I was pleased to learn that the distilling process gets rid of all the gluten. (While all distilled alcohol is gluten-free, if a flavoring agent is added after distillation there is a slight chance the product is not gluten-free. Call the manufacturer if you have questions.)

That's right, even that vodka made from wheat or whiskey made from rye is gluten-free. Some people choose to avoid it anyway, but this isn't necessary if you enjoy it. One of my favorite cocktails, an old New Orleans recipe called the Sazerac, is made with rye: two ounces rye whiskey, a dash of Angostura bitters, a quarter shot of Herbsaint (an anise-flavored liqueur), with a twist (at least, that's how I make it). Enjoy!

Read the Label

Sake, sometimes called rice wine, is a fermented beverage made from rice and koji mold (rice to which koji mold spores have been added). While koji mold can be grown on other substrates such as barley or soy, this seems unlikely for a rice-based beverage. If you have concerns about the source of koji mold used in a particular brand of sake, you should contact the distributor. For a great description of how sake is made, see the website www.sake-world.com.

Brandy Is Dandy

Okay, my rhyming section titles are getting a bit much, I realize (no, I haven't been drinking while writing this). But this one was just too easy … brandy *is* dandy because it doesn't contain gluten and it's a delicious after-dinner drink. So is cognac. Other sweet liqueurs are fine, too, like Kahlua, Irish Cream, Grand Marnier, Frangelico, Campari, Drambuie, Ouzo, and all flavors of Schnapps (there are many others). If a flavoring has been added after distillation, there is a chance (albeit slight) the product is not gluten-free. Contact the manufacturer if you have questions.

Cocktails ... With Caution

In our house, Wednesday night is "date night." Restaurants aren't crowded, and Ben and I go out, kid-free, to enjoy good service and a relaxed atmosphere. Just the other night, we went to one of our favorite restaurants—one of those nice ones that knows all about gluten-free eating and will prepare what I want in a version without gluten, using separate cookware and everything. It's very nice. But I digress.

The point is that we were sitting at the bar for an aperitif, and I was in the mood for a margarita, so I ordered one. I drank it, and it was really good. Then we started talking to the bartender about what to order, and I mentioned that I would need the food to be gluten-free and asked if he could check to see which specials of the evening could be made that way. He said he would and asked if I wanted another margarita. I said, "Sure!"

The bartender started towards the kitchen, then stopped, turned around, and said, somewhat sheepishly, "So … I shouldn't put beer in the margarita this time?"

Oops. This restaurant's "secret" margarita ingredient was a splash of beer. Despite my delicious salmon entrée without gluten, I was up at 3 A.M., sick to my stomach.

(Yes, I know, I went gluten-free to write this book and am not diagnosed with celiac disease—but I was sick anyway. Coincidence?)

My point is that even though distilled liquor doesn't contain gluten, a cocktail made with distilled liquor *could* contain gluten. So even if you feel embarrassed, even if you don't want to cause trouble, *it never hurts to ask if something has gluten,* even if you don't think it would. Who would have thought a margarita would have beer in it? If I would have been more careful, I suspect I would have had a much better night.

You can look in cocktail books for gluten-free cocktails, but again, you never know how an individual bartender might decide to make a cocktail. Plus, cocktail mixes might contain gluten, so check the label, or ask the bartender to let you see it. If you make drinks at home, check mixers. Margarita, daiquiri, piña colada, and sour mixes are likely to be gluten-free, but you can't know for sure unless you read the label.

The Least You Need to Know

- You can still drink beer if it's brewed without barley or wheat. Look for gluten-free beers made from sorghum, rice, buckwheat, and other gluten-free grains.

- Wine is fine.

- Distilled liquor is also gluten-free, even if it's made from gluten-containing grains. The distilling process removes all the gluten.

- Cocktails could contain gluten—be sure you know what's in the mix.

Part 4

Gluten-Free Dining

You *can* eat and thrive gluten-free! In this part, we reveal the best tips and secrets of gluten-free cooking so you can feel confident that the meals you make will turn out great—even without wheat. You'll learn to make substitutions that will convert recipes into gluten-free recipes—don't abandon those treasured family favorites! Plus, you'll find a core arsenal of wonderful gluten-free recipes to add to your repertoire and a whole week of gluten-free menus to get you started.

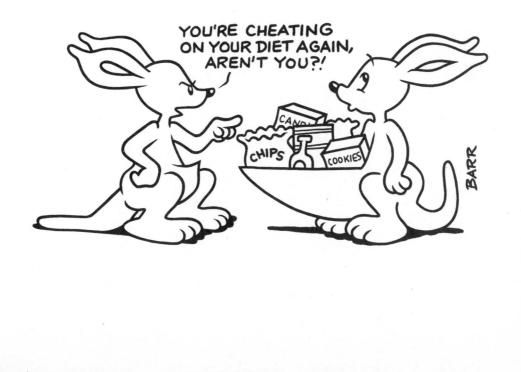

Chapter 11

Thriving in a World of Gluten

In This Chapter

◆ Coping with gluten-free eating out in the world

◆ Ways to manage the people who just don't get it

◆ Eating out at restaurants or with friends, gluten-free

◆ Handling temptation

◆ Finding the support you crave

Wow! It's tough out there!

I mean, really! Eating gluten-free is tough! I feel your pain, and I don't mean the gutache part.

And the funny thing is, it's not just tough because you wish you could eat something out of the bread basket in the restaurant or because you long for a croissant.

It's tough because of *people*.

I suppose in a perfect world, everybody would be entirely understanding and supportive of everybody else's politics, religious beliefs, and dietary restrictions. Unfortunately, however, it just ain't so. If you eat "on the fringe," whether by choice or by necessity, every now and then, people are going to give you trouble about it. Sometimes, they even act threatened by it or angry about it. Why? I really have no idea, but it's true.

In this chapter, we do our best to prepare you for some of the situations you might encounter as you live your life eating gluten-free and give you some strategies that can help you get through the day feeling good.

Family and Friends

You love them. They mean well. But the people you live with and spend the most time with can be among the most difficult obstacles to your gluten-free changeover. We all have our unique situations, but many of us deal with the same kinds of situations. Do these sound familiar?

Gluten-Free Misconceptions

Every time I cook something these days, my kids look at it suspiciously and ask, "Is this gluten-free?" If I say yes, then they are likely to say, before even tasting it, "I'm not eating this. Why should we have to eat this stuff just because you do?" Never mind that it's *delicious*, you ungrateful children! Sometimes I just snap, "Then make your own dinner!" which doesn't make for a peaceful evening.

Sometimes friends make it tough, too. Recently, we hosted a big multi-course Italian dinner party at my house, and my friend said, "You aren't going to be gluten-free *tonight*, are you? Because I have this incredible tiramisu recipe."

At restaurants now, my family and friends all give me worried looks before I order, as if to say, "You're not going to embarrass us, are you?" or "Is your order going to take a *really long time to explain?*"

The other day, at a potluck, I commented that the cake looked really good. A friend said to me, "Well, can't you just eat the frosting off the top?"

Part of the problem is that people have some misconceptions about eating gluten-free. Some people think it's just a fad diet or a dietary whim or the latest weight-loss scheme. Some people think I am just being difficult or trying to get attention. And some people can't imagine life without bread, so they don't really believe anybody could live this way.

We understand. You're tired of people rolling their eyes at you or sighing or acting inconvenienced. You're tired of people thinking you can just eat the frosting off the cake or the topping off the pizza or the tuna salad off the sandwich. You're tired of saying "no" to foods you used to love.

Now, first, remember that other people feel like this, too. You're not alone.

Second, remember that it's okay if other people don't understand your dietary restrictions. Rather than expecting others to make allowances for you (although they often will), take your health into your own hands. You're doing this for *you*. And that's great. If people try to get you to eat foods you can't eat, just say something like, "I'm sorry, I wish I could eat that but it will make me feel really ill." This works very well because nobody who cares about you wants you to feel ill, even if they don't understand why.

It's Not You, It's Me

Finally, recognize that sometimes the problem really isn't the other people. I know that for me, sometimes, quite frankly, it's *me* who's the difficult one. I'm afraid of inconveniencing people or annoying people, so I go out of my way to make it easier for others, or I just don't eat (and feel horribly deprived and dramatic about it).

Yes, the world can seem like a pretty unforgiving place when you can't always do what everybody else does. We don't always realize that others don't want us to feel bad, that people will often go out of their way to accommodate a special need, that we are lucky to have found out what the problem is and have an easy way to fix it (just by changing our entire diets … which as you and I both know by now isn't as easy as it seems), and that the people who love us want us to be healthy. Sometimes, when people aren't so accommodating, you feel all alone. Eating gluten-free suddenly seems unfair and unpleasant. On those days, how do you get through the day?

Try these strategies:

- Have a daily indulgence. Whether it's a piece of gluten-free dark chocolate or a gluten-free cookie, a leisurely stroll through the fresh air, a half-hour alone in your room with a good book, or an hour of yoga, take time for *you*. Then you won't feel so deprived.

- Remember that food is not life. When you can't eat something, it can tend to take over your mind and make you think about it all the time. Cultivate your other interests. It's just food, even if sometimes it seems like more.

- Have a support system. Relative, partner, friend, or support group, get support from others who like to talk about gluten-free eating and share inspirational ideas about it. You need people who understand what you are going through.

When you get the chance to air your grievances and share your successes with others who know what you are talking about, you'll feel much better. See the last section of this chapter for some resources.

Fearless Eater
It's really nice to have at least one person who accepts what you need to do—a partner, a sibling, or a best friend who sympathizes can make all the difference. Ben is very conscious about my gluten-free needs, and whenever we talk with others about restaurants or plan parties or just try to figure out what to have for dinner, he always says, "But can you find something to eat? Do they have something gluten-free?" He's not gluten-free, but because he always remembers that I am, it makes it much easier to tolerate all those people who seem to want to make it more difficult.

Family Members Who Won't Get Tested

One of the most frustrating things that someone diagnosed with celiac disease may encounter is the family member who won't get tested. The more I talk to people who eat gluten-free and the more I learn about it, the more stories I hear about people whose close relatives probably have celiac disease and refuse to do anything about it. This can be incredibly difficult for the person (you) who has gone through the whole process of getting diagnosed, gone gluten-free, and is enjoying incredible benefits. You can't stand to see your mother, your sister, your nephew, or even one of your own grown children continue to suffer.

We've heard about people who say they couldn't live without bread so they don't want to know. We've heard about people who refuse to believe anybody is really gluten-intolerant. We've heard about people who insist they have some other problem, even though many people in their own families have been diagnosed with celiac disease. We've even heard about family members who have decided that people who don't eat gluten are just plain crazy (as they continue to suffer from digestive problems and ill health).

These attitudes are too bad because if you have family members with celiac disease, your chances of having it are much higher than someone's chances in the general population. However, the fact is that you (probably) aren't a doctor, and while you can take your underaged children to the doctor for testing, you can't force your uncle or your brother or your grandchildren, for that matter, to get tested for celiac disease, and you certainly can't decide that they have celiac disease.

You got tested, and that's great. Even if you wish you didn't have celiac disease (and who doesn't wish that?), it's better to know and do what it takes to heal. However, you can't make that decision for anyone else.

Tempting as it is to be a gluten-free evangelist, all you can do is continue to live your life in the healthiest way possible and set a good example for others. Maybe they'll come around, but if they don't, it's not your fault.

Restaurant Options

Eating in restaurants can be so frustrating that a lot of people who eat gluten-free have simply thrown in the towel and stay home. However, some restaurants are incredibly accommodating. You really must be careful, though, to ask and make sure the chef knows you need everything prepared gluten-free without wheat, rye, barley, malt, or oats.

Sushi restaurants that prepare rolls without soy sauce are good choices. So are Mexican restaurants if you order dishes made with corn tortillas (just make sure any sauces are gluten-free). Good old-fashioned steak restaurants are good, too, if you like the whole meat-and-potatoes kind of food (just pass on the bread basket). But even if the menu item *looks* gluten-free, always ask, just to be sure, especially about sauces, seasoning mixes (like seasoned fish or any meat dredged in anything—ask because the menu might not *say* the meat is dredged, even though the chef prepares it that way), and salad dressing (and don't forget to order the salad without croutons).

For more information on eating in restaurants, see Chapter 15.

Successful Socializing

It's a party! You don't have to dread social events if you are prepared. Social events can be a real challenge because everybody is having a great time, making merry, and eating together. You don't want to spoil the fun by bringing up all your dietary restrictions or staring longingly at the dessert table while everybody else indulges. You'll just make everybody feel bad, and if you're too much trouble to invite, people might stop inviting you!

In fact, I have a strictly vegan friend who never goes to parties or out with friends because it's just too much trouble trying to explain or sitting there watching everybody else eat. But you don't have to fall victim to that fate. You can still be the life of the party *and* gluten-free. Here's how:

- Bring food! Offer to bring your own gluten-free entrée, appetizers, or whatever. And don't forget a bottle of something you can drink, too, whether it's a six-pack of gluten-free beer or a nice bottle of wine or a carafe of your famous fresh-squeezed lemonade.

- Eat before you go so you aren't starving and faced with a table full of food you can't eat. If you aren't hungry, then it won't be a big deal.

- Keep your sense of humor.

- Talk about something other than food. It's a big, interesting world out there. Why not start up a heated debate about politics? That will take everybody's mind off the fact that you aren't eating the canapés.

- Remember how your mother always used to tell you that nobody really cares what you are wearing because they are too busy worrying about what they are wearing? The same goes for what you are eating. When it comes right down to it, everybody has their own issues, and nobody really cares all that much whether you had any birthday cake.

Temptation!

Oh, but *you* might care that you didn't have any birthday cake. You might be cursing your gut for keeping you from that warm, soft loaf of bread. You might want an old-fashioned gooey chocolate chip cookie in the *worst* way. Whether you are at a social event or it's just you and a bagel staring each other down all alone at home with no witnesses, you are going to feel temptation. We can practically guarantee it.

If you get really sick after eating gluten, you have a built-in temptation buster. You *know* how you'll feel in the middle of the night, so you know it's not worth it. But what if you are one of those people who doesn't get digestive distress from eating gluten, or doesn't *always?* It's going to be easy to try to convince yourself that a little bit of this or that will be just fine; that you can eat gluten *just this once;* or that even though you *know* you shouldn't, you *know* it's not good for you, you just really really really want to eat something with gluten.

For me, it was pizza. My kids really wanted some pizza, so I ordered it for them. And then I watched them eat it … the soft puffy crust, the gooey cheese, the warm savory steamy smell of the thing … do I have to tell you how badly I wanted to eat *just one little piece? Just one little bite?*

Yep, sometimes we are our own worst enemies. I didn't give in to temptation (phew!) but at some point, I might. And maybe you might. And maybe you have. So how do you prevent that from happening?

◆ **Be a Boy Scout.** The best way to nip temptation before it nips you in the small intestine is to be prepared. Yes, just like a boy scout. When temptation hits, you need to be ready with something equally delicious that you really really love, something delicious and gluten-free. Luckily, I happened to have a Van Harden's Cheese-Crust Pizza in the freezer. The crust is made from cheese, and it has the same hot gooey taste as regular pizza, so I cooked one up and enjoyed it. And I tried not to look at the crusts the kids left on their plates.

◆ **Toss the Temptations.** At home, you can best avoid temptation by getting rid of all the gluten-filled food, but as anybody knows who lives with people who aren't gluten-free, that isn't always possible. At least try to get rid of the foods that really tempt you. If it's bagels, don't buy them. If it's pasta, get the gluten-free kind. Those wanting the semolina variety can order it when they eat out. The trick is to reorient your kitchen so that all the tempting things also happen to be gluten-free.

◆ **Never Get Too Hungry.** Away from home, you also have to be prepared. Eat before you go out; bring your own food; keep gluten-free snacks in your purse; and always be ready to face temptation with another option. If you are never totally starving, you'll be in a much better position to make a sensible decision.

◆ **Know Your Local Resources.** Cultivate your *new* favorite foods by exploring local restaurants for the best and yummiest gluten-free options. When friends say, "Where should we go out to eat?" don't say, "I don't care." Be ready! Say, "What about that new café with the great California cuisine?" or "I'm in the mood for sushi!" or "Mexican sounds great to me." If you know where to go, you won't get caught off guard.

◆ **Be a Little Food-Snobbish.** Of course, sometimes you will be caught off guard, but cultivating a little bit of food snobbery never hurt, either. If everybody is dying for pasta, order a salad (hold the croutons) or salmon and steamed vegetables or a vegetable stir-fry (hold the soy sauce), and as your friends wolf down those big plates of carbs, you can raise your eyebrows. No, you don't have to be rude. The point is to take an empowered attitude rather than a victim attitude. If you face the situation with an "I wouldn't eat that stuff if you paid me" attitude rather than an "It's so unfair you all get to eat that and I can't" attitude, you'll feel a lot better about your smart and healthy choices.

Gluten-Free Support

Even if your family won't join your gluten-free quest, even if your friends just don't get it, many, many people out there *do* get it. We're talking about gluten-free support groups, and they can be a real lifesaver for someone who feels like she is eating gluten-free in a vacuum, because nobody should have to be a gluten-free island.

Some of these groups are local and meet face-to-face every month or however often. Check with your local hospital, health resource center, health food store, local nutritionists, or ask your doctor. These people all might know of local gluten-free support groups. You might be able to strike up some new friendships with people who understand what you're going through. Or search "gluten-free support" and the name of your city on the Internet to see if anything comes up. For a listing of national support groups, see Appendix B.

Many other support groups are online—the perfect way to commune with the gluten-free side of the world without ever leaving the comfort of your home. Because I eat mostly vegetarian, I like the gluten-free vegetarian group on Yahoo!, but there are many others. Sign up, log on, introduce yourself, and get ready to make some good friends, share recipes and cooking tips, dish on the latest gluten-free products and how they taste, find out where to buy which kind of rice tortilla, which brand of pasta tastes best, and how to make a really good loaf of gluten-free bread. Commiserate with others about missing flaky piecrust or a really good, dark, malty beer. And just "hang out" with other people who eat gluten-free and know what it's like. I can't tell you how refreshing that is! To get your search started, check out these groups. Read about them and see which ones appeal to you.

Read the Label

Online support groups are usually comprised of regular people who want to chat with others and share their experiences. They are not typically populated by medical professionals, so an online support group is *not* the place to get medical advice. Instead, rely on online support groups to meet people and share lifestyle tips. As ever, be smart and careful about divulging personal information on the Internet.

Celiac.com

This huge and comprehensive gluten-free resource also has a message board where people can post questions and talk to other people who are eating gluten-free. The site also has a subscription newsletter and an online store. To find the message board and start interacting with others, go here: www.glutenfreeforum.com.

Yahoo! Groups

I always use Yahoo! so I usually look there for groups that interest me. These are some of the most popular Yahoo! gluten-free groups, but believe it or not, this isn't a complete list. Still, you're sure to find one you enjoy.

◆ Silly Yaks Online Support Group: http://health.groups.yahoo.com/group/SillyYaks

   Silly Yaks, a cute twist on "celiacs," is a general support group for anybody with celiac disease or those who live with someone who has celiac disease. It's a large group with tons of great information, including a real-time chat section and tons of great gluten-free resources like recipes, product lists, and information for chain restaurants. You can spend a lot of time here—check it out!

◆ Vegetarian & Gluten-Free (VGF) Group: http://groups.yahoo.com/group/vegetariangf

   This is my favorite group, and I really enjoy "hanging out" here. I've gotten great tips on vegetarian products without gluten and passed on some tips, too. I've gotten some great recipes and general moral support, too. Some people eat dairy and/or eggs on this list, and some are totally vegan (strict vegetarian with no animal products of any kind).

◆ Gluten-Free Kitchen: http://health.groups.yahoo.com/group/glutenfreekitchen

   Put on your apron and get ready to cook … and talk about cooking. This is an interactive mailing list with information and recipes.

◆ Gluten-Free Casein-Free Recipes (GFCFrecipes): http://health.groups.yahoo.com/group/GFCFrecipes

   This group focuses on gluten-free and casein-free recipes, specifically geared toward parents of kids who follow this type of diet.

◆ Food Allergy Kitchen: http://groups.yahoo.com/group/FOODALLERGYKITCHEN

   This group is a recipe exchange group for people with all kinds of food allergy issues, from wheat allergies to dairy allergies to peanut allergies. They also cover gluten-free eating, vegetarianism, and other special diets.

◆ Vegan and Gluten-Free: http://groups.yahoo.com/group/Vegan-and-Gluten-Free

For the strict vegetarian who doesn't eat any animal products including milk, eggs, or even honey, here you'll find tons of great information about vegan and gluten-free eating. Eating gluten-free and vegan is easier than you thought!

CELIAC Listserve

This link allows you to sign up for the Celiac listserve which has over 3,000 members in 33 countries who chat about gluten-free eating. You can also find links to Cel-Kids, a list for kids with celiac disease, Cel-Pro for medical professionals, Celiac-Dietetic for dietitians, Celiac-Diabetes for people who also have diabetes, and Cel-Gps for support group leader support. Check it out here: www.enabling.org/ia/celiac.

The Least You Need to Know

◆ Family and friends won't always understand your diet, and that's okay.

◆ Manage social situations and eating out by knowing your options and never showing up to an event too hungry.

◆ Gluten-filled foods may tempt you, but being prepared with alternatives, and changing your attitude if necessary, can help ward off a slip-up.

◆ Many gluten-free support groups exist that can provide you with practical and emotional support as well as new friends who know exactly what it's like to eat gluten-free.

The Secret of a Gluten-Free Chef: Substitution

- ◆ Gluten-free cooking: what it's all about
- ◆ A new look at old favorites
- ◆ Baking secrets for sweet success
- ◆ Gluten-free gourmet cooking

I love to cook, and I usually don't like to use a recipe. I like to make it up as I go along … a little of this, a little of that, a taste, an adjustment, a little more of this, a dash of that, and voilà! Dinner.

But now that I'm eating gluten-free, cooking in my kitchen isn't quite the free-for-all it once was. I have to be much more careful. I can't just thicken that sauce with a roux or whip up muffins with that bag of unbleached flour or dump a bottle of beer in the chili anymore.

However, cooking gluten-free has also made me more creative. How might arrowroot work in that sauce? What about baking muffins with a mixture of brown rice flour and potato starch? And what about a white chili with diced chicken breast, white beans, green chilies, and a dash of sauvignon blanc instead of beer? (Everybody loved it.)

In this chapter, we let you in on a few secrets we've learned while cooking gluten-free in our own homes. Even if you don't like to cook, you'll get some basic direction to help you prepare gluten-free foods in the easiest possible way. You just need the right ingredients. If you do like to cook, this chapter can be your springboard into a world of gluten-free cuisine. Gluten-free gourmet? Absolutely!

Substitutions ... and Beyond!

We can break gluten-free cooking into two basic concepts:

1. You can make just about anything you made before you began eating gluten-free if you know what ingredients to substitute for the gluten-containing ingredients you used to use.

2. You can open up a whole new world of cuisine by exploring foods that never contained gluten in the first place.

Gluten-free eating seems a lot less limiting once you begin cooking and discovering how much you really can make. You can bake, make pasta dishes, and thicken gravy. Making these dishes is mostly just a matter of finding other things to use in place of the wheat, rye, or barley you have been using.

But you can also stretch your mind beyond your typical cereal-for-breakfast, sandwich-for-lunch, pasta-for-dinner mentality. Consider the potential of salads, homemade soup, one-pot meals, stir-fry, and the use of delicious alternative grains like quinoa, buckwheat, and amaranth that don't have to be a substitute for anything. The world is full of fascinating foods and flavor combinations that have nothing to do with wheat, rye, and barley. This is your chance to really spread those culinary wings.

Fearless Eater

The first time I really craved spaghetti after going gluten-free, I knew I was going to have to get creative. That's when I discovered the versatility of rice noodles! I cooked up some Chinese rice noodles (ingredients: rice, water), then tossed them with a little sesame oil, chopped green onions, and sesame seeds. Along with a big salad, I found it to be a very satisfying dinner. You could also add a broiled chicken breast or salmon filet if you like.

But many of us feel a lot more comfortable in the kitchen if we can work on familiar ground, so let's start by looking at the best ways to transform some of those staples in the American diet.

Transforming Old Favorites

If breakfast to you has always meant toast or dinner has always involved some kind of pasta or bread, you can keep on eating mostly the way you have been as long as you make some adjustments. Most obviously, you can just substitute purchased gluten-free versions of the foods you were eating before, like pasta made from rice or quinoa, corn tortillas instead of flour, and gluten-free packaged bread, gravy, pretzels, etc. (see Chapter 9 and Appendix B for gluten-free packaged food resources). You can use these basics to cook with, too, when you need bread crumbs, for example, or something to wrap up refried beans and cheese.

But nothing tastes quite as good as home-made, and whether you're crazy about cooking or not, you will appreciate the fresh flavor and personal touch when you cook it yourself.

But don't ditch your old recipes just yet! First, check out these tips for transforming your old favorites into gluten-free sensations. Your family may not even notice. (And you might find you've improved on some of those family recipes.)

Good for You

Delicious gluten-free meals you probably already cook and enjoy:

- Chili with corn chips
- Stir-fry over rice
- Enchiladas, tostados, quesadillas, and other Mexican meals made with corn tortillas
- Steak and potatoes
- Chicken soup with rice
- Chef's salad

- **Coat it.** If you have to coat something in breading, use gluten-free breadcrumbs or crumbled tortilla chips, corn meal, or even crunched-up gluten-free cereal. Chicken breasts, fish filets, and sticks of drained tofu work great this way—just dip them in beaten egg, milk, or soy milk, then dredge them in the crumbs. Bake as usual. My kids love 'em.

- **Thicken it.** If you need to thicken something like gravy or sauce, use arrowroot, tapioca starch, or cornstarch instead of wheat flour. You can have your Hollandaise and eat it, too.

- **Explore pasta alternatives.** You can make all your old recipes for spaghetti, lasagna, macaroni and cheese, and more, but you may have to experiment a little to find gluten-free pastas you like. I've grown to be quite fond of several different kinds of rice noodles, rice spaghetti, quinoa spaghetti, and other shapes of pasta, particularly Tinkyada brand.

◆ **Go topless.** Instead of using bread for sandwiches, go topless. Spread or layer sandwich filling on toasted corn tortillas or rice cakes for open-faced flavor. No top is required. Or just dip tortilla chips in that batch of egg salad. It's one of my favorite lunches. Delicious!

◆ **Slam-drunk sides.** Replace that loaf of bread or those dinner rolls you're so used to having at dinner as a side dish with more creative options. Try a quinoa pilaf, slices of fried polenta, creamy risotto, or warm corn tortillas with butter.

◆ **Become a soup specialist, a salad savant.** Soups and salads don't need gluten, and provide a palette for endless creativity. Use what's fresh and in-season or whatever you have on hand. Throw it together with broth for soup (check the label to be sure the broth is gluten-free) or fresh greens for salad, and you've got a light meal.

◆ **Create one-pot meals.** Long live the one-pot meal! Like soup and salad, one-pot meals can provide endless possibilities for invention. Layer beans, meat, or cheese with your favorite veggies and torn-up corn tortillas, rice, or gluten-free pasta. For recipe ideas, see Chapter 13.

Fearless Eater

One of my favorite one-pot meals is so easy, it hardly even needs a recipe. Tear up corn tortillas and put them in the bottom of a baking dish; layer with black beans, shredded cheese, chopped tomatoes, diced green chilies (or any leftovers you have); then repeat the layers. End with a third layer of tortillas and cheese. Pour four eggs mixed with half a cup milk over the whole thing, season with salt and pepper, and bake in a 375° oven until the custard is set. Serve with your favorite salsa—great for *any* meal.

Baking Tips

Gluten-free baking is fun, but it can also be tricky. You can throw whatever you have in the vegetable bin into a soup, but you can't just bake with ingredients willy-nilly, or those muffins, cookies, or quick breads aren't going to turn out right.

Part of the reason for this unfortunate fact is that baking has to be more precise in general to effect that perfect texture. You've got complex chemical processes at work here. But a big part of the challenge that comes with gluten-free baking is just that: the absence of gluten. Gluten is the very element in wheat flour that holds things together and gives baked goods that springy texture. It lets you throw pizza crust into the air without splattering all over the walls. It helps bread rise, gives cookies their chewy texture, and makes cakes springy. Without it, things get crumbly and tend to fall apart.

That means that when you bake, you need to find something to replace the gluten. You can substitute rice flour or a combination of gluten-free flours for a tender crumb, but you still might find things just don't hold together.

Some people like to use xanthan gum or guar gum as a binder. These typically come in powder form, and mixing a little in with the flour will help hold things together in much the same way gluten does. It took me a long time to break down and try this because that packet of xanthan gum cost $10! However, when I did, it was like a miracle—my homemade bread tasted like bread. My cookies didn't fall apart. My muffins didn't melt. Xanthan gum mimics the action of gluten in baking, so although baking without it can be a fun and interesting (and sometimes disastrous) challenge, baking with it is a whole lot easier. As for flours, you can choose from white rice flour, brown rice flour, potato starch, millet flour, bean flour (including soy flour), tapioca flour, arrowroot, and more. You'll probably find other options in your grocery or natural foods store, but I'm just going by what I have in my pantry right now.

> **Fearless Eater**
>
> I like to mix equal parts white rice flour, potato starch, tapioca flour, and millet flour. In fact, I just made a batch of chocolate chip muffins using this mix. They were delicious. My kids and my son's cockatiel agreed (we didn't give the cockatiel any of the chocolate chips, in case you were worried). This isn't the only flour mix I use—I like to experiment—but this one worked well for the cookies. You could substitute any whole-grain or bean flour for the millet flour, such as brown rice flour, soy flour, or wholegrain corn flour. Each has a subtly different taste.

When you don't have the right ingredients, you can always use a gluten-free baking mix. I keep one in the house at all times. I like Pamela's pancake and waffle mix, which has the baking powder already added in, and also Pamela's wheat-free bread mix, which comes with yeast (for bread, pizza crust, dinner rolls, etc.), for those days when I just don't feel like experimenting.

For specific recipes, see Chapter 13.

Go Gourmet, Gluten-Free

I have to admit I'm a foodie, but the strangest kind. I love to try exotic cuisine, and I always appreciate the efforts of a really good chef. But I also love the challenge of gourmet cuisine that pushes the limits or proves it can leave something out—whether it's meat, dairy, or gluten (or all of the above!).

If you love gourmet food, too, you'll be pleased to know you don't have to give it up to go gluten-free. In fact, the current trend in gourmet cooking seems to have left wheat flour largely by the wayside. It's *so* twentieth century.

Just flipping through a recent issue of one of my many cooking magazines (I won't even tell you how many subscriptions I have), I see some impressive, delicious-sounding recipes that just happen to be gluten-free (if you're dying to see these recipes, check out the April 2007 issue of *Saveur*):

- Stewed okra and tomatoes
- Buckwheat crepes (made with 100 percent buckwheat flour)
- Scallops in white wine cream sauce (the sauce is thickened with cornstarch)
- Cider-spiked onion confit (flavored with hard cider)
- Chive and goat cheese omelette
- Seared tri-tip sirloin steaks with chive butter
- Knife-and-fork egg salad (you can serve it on bread but the recipe also says it's delicious on its own)
- Stir-fried bean sprouts
- Ginger milk tea
- Shrimp and pineapple curry
- Coconut jam
- Braised chicken with coriander (make sure you use gluten-free soy sauce)
- Greek-style vegetables

A cursory flip through the March 2007 issue of *Food and Wine* revealed recipes that just happen to be gluten-free, by these culinary TV stars:

- Pan-roasted salmon with tomato vinaigrette (Ted Allen's recipe)
- One-pan chicken, sausage, and sage bake (Nigella Lawson's recipe)
- Green curry chicken (Nigel Slater's recipe)

- T-bone fiorentina with sautéed spinach (Mario Batali's recipe)

- Swordfish spiedini (Giada de Laurentiis' recipe)

And a Tex-Mex menu where every single item except a cookie at the end is gluten-free (and after a meal like this, who would have room for cookies?):

- Citrus and avocado salad with honey vinaigrette

- Grilled steaks with ancho mole sauce

- Two-cheese enchiladas

- Salsa roja

- Sautéed chickpeas with ham and kale

- Vanilla tapioca pudding

And in a recent issue of *Vegetarian Times* (February 2007), even more:

- Cajun-style chipotle jambalaya

- Dark-chocolate nuggets

- Chocolate crème caramel

- Divinely dairy-free chocolate coins

- Broccoli raab with pine nuts and golden raisins

- Indonesian tofu-peanut fondue

- Guadalajaran Swiss chard quesadillas

- Maple walnut polenta pudding

- Caponata stew

- Hummus cakes

- Moroccan carrot salad

- Yogurt crème with grapefruit-marsala sauce

- Crispy five-spice tofu with black bean relish

- Baby bok choy with Chinese mushrooms

- Mashed sweet potatoes with goji berries

- Spinach and red mustard salad with chickpea dal

- Snow pea and soba noodle salad with Thai peanut sauce (choose 100 percent buckwheat soba noodles)

- Millet-stuffed portobello mushrooms

- Quinoa curry

- Hearty grain soup with beans and greens (the grain in question is kasha, or buckwheat)

- Mozzarella-stuffed arancini (Italian rice balls)

- Tortilla and tomato soup

Fearless Eater

In the list of recipes from *Vegetarian Times* in this chapter, I admit (shameless self-promotion) that I wrote the recipes for Caponata stew, Hummus cakes, Moroccan carrot salad, and Yogurt crème with grapefruit-marsala sauce, for an article titled "Mediterranean Makeover." Interestingly, I didn't even intend for these to be gluten-free at the time, but yet, here they are! Meanwhile, look for my Gluten-Free Vegetarian article in the October 2007 issue of *Vegetarian Times*, which includes more recipes.

And that doesn't even mention all the rest of the recipes in both magazines that could easily be made by substituting, for example, rice pasta for regular pasta, gluten-free breadcrumbs for regular bread crumbs, and gluten-free flours for regular flour.

The point is, you can still have a great time cooking exotic gourmet creations with barely a blink in your normal routine. In fact, I would even argue that gourmet cooking is the *best* way to eat gluten-free because you are thinking outside the box, beyond the old standards of bread and pasta and pizza crust.

Gourmet cooking borrows flavors and ideas from other cultures where wheat isn't nearly so influential and combines the best and freshest ingredients in new ways. Everybody knows what wheat tastes like. Gourmet cooking allows you to go above and beyond … leaving the gluten far behind.

So now that we have you good and hungry, head straight to Chapter 13 for some of our own favorite gluten-free recipes. You'll be a gluten-free chef in no time!

The Least You Need to Know

◆ Cooking gluten-free is easy if you know what ingredients to substitute for wheat flour and other gluten-containing ingredients.

◆ Make over your old favorites by using alternative flours, alternative-grain pastas, gluten-free chips or cereal for breading, and rice cakes and corn tortillas in place of sandwich bread.

◆ Gluten-free baking is more science than art, but with the right combination of flours and binding ingredients, your muffins, cakes, and cookies will come out just fine.

◆ Gluten-free gourmet cooking is easy because it uses so many new flavors, alternative ingredients, and ethnic influences. Gluten almost becomes a nonissue.

Your Arsenal of Gluten-Free Basic Recipes

In This Chapter

◆ Staples to keep in your pantry

◆ A baking mix you can use again and again

◆ One-pot meals with personality

◆ Jazz up your meals with great side dishes

If you love to cook, bake, snack, or, quite frankly, *eat*, then you'll love this chapter, although calling it a "recipe" chapter might be a little bit, well, grand. This is more like a "get cooking" chapter, with a pantry list and some basic free-form recipes that can get you started with whatever *you* want to make. For more extensive recipes, see Appendix C for a gluten-free mini cookbook.

For now, these basic formulas will take you anywhere: a baking mix you can turn into everything from pancakes to chocolate chip cookies; a one-pot meal perfectly suited for using up leftovers that just happens to be perfect for family dinners or, with a few adjustments, a fancy dinner party; and a kid-friendly recipe for macaroni and cheese (actually, I ate most of it myself), and more. Although these recipes include dairy, I've also included dairy-free alternatives for those who can't stomach dairy products, or who choose not to eat them.

The trick to gluten-free cooking is to have some basic solutions to the problems you'll typically encounter in baking, sauce-making, thickening, and just finding something satisfying for dinner. This chapter to the rescue! Are you ready to get cooking? So are we!

Staples for Your Pantry

You can't cook gluten-free if you don't have the basic ingredients, but with a well-stocked pantry, you'll never be without something good to eat. So fill your pantry with these gluten-free basics that will make all these recipes (and your own creations) possible:

Baking supplies

- ◆ Gluten-free flour. Rice flour is probably the easiest to find. Check your Asian grocery to see if it's cheaper there than in the gluten-free section of your grocery store or the health food store. You might want to try a selection of flours, or just stick with one if you think you won't use others or don't want to pay the sometimes-hefty price tag. Personally, I keep white rice flour, brown rice flour, amaranth flour, millet flour, and soy flour on hand most of the time.

Read the Label

Don't buy gluten-free flour from bulk bins because of the potential for cross-contamination. Those scoops don't always stay in the "right" bin!

- ◆ Gluten-free starches. I keep potato starch, tapioca starch, and corn starch on hand most of the time, but if you can only find corn starch, that should be fine.

- ◆ Cornmeal. It's not only good as a hot cereal but for making polenta and gluten-free cornbread.

- ◆ Xanthan gum. Many gluten-free cooks use this in baked goods, and I resisted it for a long time, but now that I've tried it, I have to say I'm hooked. It really helps thinks stay together. It's very expensive, though, so you have our permission to consider this an optional ingredient.

- ◆ Applesauce. Here's another great baking secret for holding gluten-free baked foods together.

◆ Sugar. I try not to use white sugar very often. I find that brown sugar, raw sugar, real maple syrup, and molasses really stand in just fine for the white stuff. But if you prefer it in your baking, white sugar works fine.

◆ Molasses, real maple syrup, and honey. (See above.)

◆ Baking soda.

◆ Baking powder.

◆ Salt. I prefer sea salt and kosher salt, for better taste.

◆ Butter or margarine. Butter always tastes better, but for those who can't or don't eat dairy products, you can now buy some pretty good non-hydrogenated margarines (that means they don't contain any of that nasty trans-fat). I like Smart Balance. Tricia says to avoid margarines containing trans fats *at all costs!* She's a nutritionist, so you should listen to her.

◆ Canola oil. This is the best oil for baking because it has very little taste so it doesn't get in the way of the other flavors.

◆ Apple cider vinegar and white vinegar, distilled.

◆ Flavorings: vanilla, almond extract, etc. Read the label to be sure they are gluten-free, but most natural and artificial flavorings are. Also, don't worry about the alcohol, which is distilled. It won't contain gluten.

◆ Spices: cinnamon, nutmeg, cloves, ginger.

◆ Raisins or currants, dried cherries, dates and figs. Make sure the dates aren't dusted with gluten-containing flour—check the label.

◆ Chocolate chips, nuts, and other yummy things you like to add to cookies and muffins. Check to be sure they are gluten-free.

Dinner staples

◆ Gluten-free pasta. I always have some Tinkyada rice penne and some form of rice or quinoa spaghetti.

◆ Brown and white rice (I like basmati).

◆ Quinoa. Use it in place of rice, bulgar, or any other cooked savory grain.

◆ Gluten-free chicken and/or vegetable stock or broth. Use this to prepare rice and quinoa or for making soup.

◆ Fresh fruits and vegetables. Keep lots; they're good for you! I always have lots of fresh lemons and limes because they can flavor so many things, from fish to fruit to salad dressing.

◆ Dried legumes. Lentils, black beans, pinto beans, split peas. I usually have at least some of these around—they take longer to soak and cook but they are very economical.

◆ Canned beans. Rinse canned beans before using, to get some of that excess salt off.

◆ Frozen fruits and frozen vegetables. They provide off-season nutrition. Just make sure they are the plain variety, or if not, that they don't contain gluten.

◆ Canned crushed tomatoes. Use for chili and sauces.

◆ Eggs. I think the free-range kind taste better, but maybe it's just my imagination. Or you can use egg substitutes, like Ener-G egg replacer, if you don't eat eggs. Or use $1/4$ cup applesauce, half a mashed banana, $1/4$ cup soy yogurt, or 2 table-spoons of ground flaxseed mixed with $1/4$ cup water, set to soak until it reaches egg-white consistency. These can all stand in for an egg.

◆ Milk—skim or 1 percent cow's milk, soy milk, goat's milk, rice milk, or whatever you like. Just be sure the soy, rice, or any other nondairy milk doesn't contain gluten—I don't really see why it's necessary, but a lot of them actually do. Also, Tricia says to choose calcium and vitamin D fortified versions.

◆ Sour cream and/or yogurt. Regular, goat, soy … whatever you fancy. Tricia says to choose low-fat or nonfat versions of yogurt.

◆ Cheese. I like to have some shredded cheese around for nachos and macaroni and cheese, plus some imported goat cheese for (gluten-free) crackers and salads, when I feel like getting fancy (or just want something tangy). I also usually have low-fat cottage cheese and low-fat cream cheese. Most of these things come in soy versions. Tricia wants to remind us all to choose low-fat cheese as often as possible! Save your full-fat cheese allotment for the good French stuff.

◆ Meat, poultry, and fish. Of course, stock these only if you eat them, and choose plain, fresh, preferably organic or local versions, not those highly processed, sauce-covered, basting-solution-injected kinds, which could have gluten, and definitely have way too much salt.

◆ Corn tortillas, plain.

◆ Corn chips. These are not only good for snacks but, when crumbled, are also handy to use as breading for homemade fish sticks and other recipes that call for coating. I usually get the baked kind, just to keep the fat content to a minimum. Or you can make your own by cutting corn tortillas in wedges and baking them until crispy—no fat required!

◆ Ready-to-eat gluten-free cereal. Cereal also works as a coating.

◆ Herbs and spices to keeping things flavorful—experiment with fresh and dried herbs and whole spices you grind yourself.

You can probably think of more things, but I usually have these basics around. I usually have some gluten-free convenience foods, too, for those times when I don't feel like cooking, though in my opinion, they're too pricey and processed for eating every day.

Baking Basics

Gluten-free baking can be tricky because without the exact proportions, things won't turn out right. For example, I was testing chocolate chip cookies just this morning. My first batch ran all over the cookie sheet so that it came out looking like one giant misshapen cookie disaster. (However, it *tasted* good!) I was making up the recipe, and that's tricky to do when baking. I finally got it right—see the recipe later in this chapter.

When baking, you *can* substitute rice flour, soy flour, millet flour, amaranth, or any other gluten-free flour for wheat flour, but you will probably have to add an extra egg or more egg substitute, or something else to replace the egg (see the list earlier in this chapter about egg substitutes). The thing about baking (gluten-free or not) is that everything you substitute for anything else can change the results—either slightly, or drastically. Your chewy cookies might turn cakey. Your fluffy banana bread might turn dense. Your super-moist pancakes may turn dry or fall apart when you flip them. Or you might try something new and it makes the recipes a hundred times better than before! (This is why I think cooking is so much fun).

Anyway, my point is, you will develop your own style, discover your own secrets, invent your own dishes everybody loves … eventually. Until then, using tried-and-true recipes from good gluten-free cookbooks can be your training ground. For a list of gluten-free cookbooks and websites with gluten-free recipes, see Appendix B. And try the recipes in this chapter, too, to see how they work for you. (And don't be afraid to experiment!)

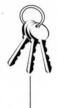

Good for You

Some people prefer the texture and nutrition of brown rice flour and other whole-grain flours, like whole-grain millet flour, to white rice flour, which can be a little fine and delicate. But for some recipes, fine and delicate is just what you want. Try different combinations to see what works for you, but remember: whole grain flours *always* have better nutrition than refined flours, gluten-free or not.

You can use a good gluten-free baking mix (like Pamela's or many others), or you can make your own. This is the one I use again and again at home, and the one I use in the other baking recipes in this book. This is different than the flour mix in Chapter 12. This one has baking powder, soda, salt, and xanthan gum, so it's all ready to go for pancakes, cookies, and quick breads.

I also put ground flaxseed in my baking mix, not only because it has healthy omega-3 fatty acids we all need, but because when it gets wet, it becomes egglike in texture and serves as a binder. It can have a strong taste, though, so don't overdo the flaxseed, especially in more delicate, light-tasting recipes.

A note about xanthan gum: if you can't find it or don't want to use it, your recipes may not stay together as well, depending on what you are making and what else you put in there. However, pancakes and muffins (especially containing bananas and/or applesauce) should be just fine without it (and also good with it). Cookies, bread, and other items that have to hold their shape don't work as well without the xanthan gum. But if you like to live dangerously, go ahead and leave it out!

Eve's Gluten-Free Baking Mix

A good basic mix for pancakes, cookies, or quickbread.

1 cup white rice flour	1 tablespoon baking powder
1 cup brown rice flour	1 teaspoon baking soda
$^1/_2$ cup starch (potato, tapioca, or corn starch)	1 teaspoon salt
	1 teaspoon xanthan gum
$^1/_4$ cup ground flaxseed	

Stir and/or sift together thoroughly. Store in an airtight container.

Chocolate Chip Cookies

I have two problems with chocolate chip cookies: One, they are usually way too sweet and fatty. Two, recipes usually make a gazillion cookies! Who needs a gazillion cookies? Packaged cookies come in sensible amounts, like 8 or 12. So I decided to make a recipe that only made two sheets worth—like buying two packages of cookies. Some to eat, some to save for tomorrow or give to your neighbor (or, if you're like me, all the neighbor kids who hang out at your house). That way, they won't sit around for days getting stale or tempting you.

It took a few tries to get this recipe right. Too much butter made them run all over the cookie sheet like a giant cookie blob. Too little made them taste like sand. Finally I decided to try a version using a little non-hydrogenated margarine (the kind with no trans fat) and applesauce. Not only are these cookies delicious, not too sweet, and mighty chocolately, but they are downright nutritious—walnuts, flaxseed from the baking mix, fruit, and deep bittersweet chocolate (you've heard the news about all those antioxidants in dark chocolate, right? I *love* that!). These won't make you feel guilty, but they will make you feel very good.

You can refrigerate the batter for up to an hour or two before baking, but it isn't necessary. The low fat content keeps these cookies in the nice round shapes you intend. These are also delicate with a cakey texture, and smaller ones are less likely to fall apart than big ones, so drop them by teaspoonfuls. If you really can't get them to stay together or don't even want to try, you can also bake these in a 9×13 baking pan for thin bar cookies, or in a 9×9 square pan for thicker ones.

You could also substitute any nut for the walnuts and any dried fruit for the chocolate chips.

Chocolate Chip Cookies

These cookies are chewy, soft, and delicate.

Makes about 24 cookies

1¹/₂ cups Eve's Gluten-Free Baking Mix

¹/₂ teaspoon cinnamon

¹/₃ cup non-hydrogentated margarine (I use Smart Balance)

¹/₃ cup raw sugar

¹/₃ cup molasses

¹/₂ cup applesauce

¹/₂ cup bittersweet chocolate chips (gluten-free of course)

¹/₂ cup chopped walnuts

Preheat the oven to 375°.

In a small bowl, combine gluten-free baking mix and cinnamon. Stir with a fork until completely incorporated.

In another bowl, combine margarine, sugar, and molasses. Beat until well combined. Scrape down the sides of the bowl with rubber spatula. Add the dry mixture in three parts, alternating with the applesauce in two parts. (Start and end with the dry mixture.) Beat after each addition. Stir in chocolate chips and walnuts.

Lightly grease a cookie sheet or spray with gluten-free cooking spray. Drop the batter by teaspoonfuls about 2 inches apart. (I use one of those mini ice cream scoops for even, round cookies.) Bake for ten minutes. Allow to cool for ten minutes, then remove from the cookie sheet carefully (they are fragile), using a metal spatula for best results. Cool on a wire rack.

Enjoy warm, or store in an airtight container when cool.

Good for You

If your cookies break into pieces because you made them too big or didn't use a sharp spatula to get them off the sheet or it's just one of those days, don't despair! Crumble them in layers with yogurt for trifle or press them into the bottom of a pie plate and fill with pudding or yogurt (gluten-free of course) and refrigerate for an hour or two, for a quick and easy pie. Or make bar cookies.

Blueberry Pancakes

Pancakes can be so delicious—or they can turn out rubbery, dry, or flavorless. The key is a good mix, so use a gluten-free baking mix for your pancake experiments. Or try the recipe below using the baking mix in this chapter.

Blueberry Pancakes

These pancakes are tender, fruity, and quick to make with baking mix.

1 cup Eve's Gluten-Free Baking Mix

2 tablespoons brown sugar

$^1/_2$ teaspoon cinnamon

$^1/_4$ teaspoon nutmeg

1 tablespoon ground flaxseed mixed with 3 tablespoons hot water (let sit for 10 minutes), or 1 egg (if you use the flax method instead of the egg, this is in addition to the ground flax already in the baking mix)

1 cup milk (regular or soy)

1 tablespoon canola oil

1 teaspoon vanilla

$^1/_2$ cup fresh or frozen blueberries

Combine flour mixture, brown sugar, cinnamon, and nutmeg in a large bowl.

In a separate bowl, combine the flaxseed mixture or egg, milk, oil, and vanilla. Add to dry ingredients and stir just until combined (it can be a little lumpy).

Put a little canola oil or gluten-free cooking spray into a skillet and heat to medium-high. Pour pancakes in and sprinkle each with blueberries. When edges start to bubble, flip pancakes and cook an additional one minute. Serve with real maple syrup and a handful of chopped nuts or a dollop of vanilla yogurt.

Fearless Eater
I add so many different things to pancakes, depending on what I have available. Try walnuts and raisins, dried cherries and almonds, chopped strawberries and bananas, or chocolate chips. Are you thinking, "Does she put chocolate chips in *everything?*" Yes. Yes, I do.

Banana Bread

This moist yummy bread makes a great breakfast or afternoon snack with coffee or tea. I like this with cherries and sliced almonds, but it's also delicious with snipped dried apricots and pecans or currents and walnuts. Any other dried fruit/nut combination that sounds good to you would work, too.

Banana Bread

Moist and tender, dense and lush, this banana bread makes a great breakfast.

2 cups mashed ripe bananas (about 3 bananas)	**1 tablespoon vanilla**
$^1/_2$ cup brown sugar	**2 cups Eve's Gluten-Free Baking Mix**
$^1/_2$ cup maple syrup	**$^1/_2$ cup dried cherries (or other dried fruit)**
$^1/_2$ cup canola oil	
1 cup unsweetened applesauce	**$^1/_2$ cup sliced almonds (or other chopped nuts)**

Preheat oven to 325°.

In a large mixing bowl, place bananas, sugar, syrup, oil, applesauce, and vanilla. Stir and mix until the mixture looks uniform (banana lumps are just fine).

Stir in baking mix, dried fruit, and nuts. Pour into a greased loaf pan. Bake for about 70 minutes, or until deep golden brown. A toothpick may come out with moist crumbs, but if it comes out with batter on it, bake it a little longer.

Allow to cool for about an hour before removing from the pan. Or take out a slice while still in the pan if you like it warm with butter. Tastes great the next day, too.

What's for Dinner?

Figuring out what to eat for dinner is always a challenge, even for people who don't eat gluten-free, but a few good recipes can take all the hemming and hawing out of meal planning. Start with these yummy ideas, and you'll have the whole family complementing your cooking skill and asking for seconds.

One-Pot, Everything Good

I call this One-Pot, Everything Good because it can have anything you like in it— anything gluten-free, that is. (I would call it a casserole—I love casseroles!—but Tricia doesn't like the old-time association with that word, which conjures visions of "mystery meat" and tasteless leftovers for many people. If you don't mind the word, you can call it a casserole.) You just change out the different categories according to what you have, what's fresh and in-season, or whatever strikes your fancy, and voilà! You've got a meal that serves six to eight people. Try it! (Note that all elements are generally precooked, making this a great way to use leftovers—even if you don't call it a casserole!)

The great thing about this meal is that you can not only vary the ingredients but also vary the order in which you use them, the amounts, and the flavorings. Add more sauce; double the spices; stir in some plain low-fat yogurt; or whatever. Double this or cut the amounts in half or even in fourths. Do what you want; I promise not to be offended. It's *your* One-Pot, Everything Good dinner.

By the way, you can also make this in the crock-pot. Cook on low all day or high for about four hours. Or, for an even quicker meal, mix it all together in a big pot on the stove.

> **Fearless Eater**
>
> If you make one-pot meals every few days, you'll cut way down on the amount of leftover food you throw away. Talk about thrifty! Nothing makes you feel environmentally and financially responsible like actually eating all your leftovers. (Or maybe that's just me.)

One-Pot, Everything Good

Savory, filling, and ultimately versatile, this dish has your favorite grains, meat, veggies, and sauce—and it can be different every time.

4 cups of any cooked gluten-free grains, such as brown rice or quinoa

2 cups of any gluten-free cooked protein sources, such as leftover chicken breast cut into bite-size pieces, cooked flaked salmon, or a can of black beans, drained and rinsed

2 cups chopped vegetables, whatever is in the refrigerator or in season

1 cup sauce, salsa, gluten-free spaghetti sauce, or white sauce (see recipe for Flexible Sauce later in this chapter)

Preheat the oven to 375°.

Spray a casserole dish with gluten-free nonstick cooking spray. Put in half the grains, then chicken, salmon, or beans, vegetables, and remaining grains. Pour sauce over the top. If you like, sprinkle on a little cheese, salsa, or your favorite herbs and spices.

Bake for one hour or until heated through.

Good for You

Your cooking will be extra flavorful and interesting if you grow your own herbs, and it's fun, too. You'll have a little bit of nature all for you. It's easy to set up a container garden of your favorite fresh herbs. Keep it out on your deck or porch during the summer or in a sunny window. I harvest cilantro and basil out of mine all summer long, replanting the cilantro every few weeks so I get a continuous crop because I make a *lot* of salsa, pico de gallo, and guacamole.

Flexible Sauce

Sauces add interest to lots of foods, whether you want pasta in cheese sauce or fettuccine alfredo or just want to liven up your vegetables. Use this base, and add herbs, cheese, or whatever.

Flexible Sauce

The basic white sauce can go in any direction, flavored with herbs, cheese, spice, or whatever you like.

2 tablespoons butter

1 tablespoon potato or corn starch

1 cup skim or 1 percent milk or gluten-free soy or rice milk

$^1\!/_2$ teaspoon salt

Melt butter in medium saucepan over medium heat. Add starch and stir until completely combined. In a slow drizzle, add milk, stirring constantly. Keep stirring until sauce boils, which could take up to ten minutes. Add salt and let it bubble for one minute, add the salt, then add any of the following:

- ◆ 1 cup shredded cheese (cut the fat by using low-fat cheese)
- ◆ 1 tablespoon fresh herbs
- ◆ 1 teaspoon dried herbs
- ◆ Dash of gluten-free soy sauce, hot sauce, or barbecue sauce

Macaroni and Cheese

My kids love this. Heck, *I* love this. What's not to love about pasta and cheese? I don't care for soy cheese in this recipe, but you might like it. Or try low-fat cheese to lighten it. If you don't eat dairy, just cook the macaroni with the white sauce made with soy milk, or just layer in your favorite sautéed veggies. I particularly recommend mushrooms.

You can jazz this up a lot. Add a cup of salsa and cover it with crumbled tortilla chips before baking. Add the ingredients from your leftover stir-fry, put in a few dashes of gluten-free tamari sauce, and sprinkle with chopped green onions. Fill it with whatever chopped vegetables you bought at the farmer's market that day, steamed or sautéed with a little olive oil. Or just serve it plain—it's the only way my picky-eater 9-year-old will even consider it. (He'll have his veggies on the side—raw, plain, and not touching any other food, thank you very much!) This looks fattening, but it serves eight, so just have a little. Tricia recommends using low-fat cheese, and it tastes just great in this recipe.

Macaroni and Cheese

Rich, creamy, and filling with tender pasta and cheese sauce.

1 pound rice pasta (I use Tinkyada penne.)

1 recipe Flexible Sauce with shredded cheese (I use a low-fat cheddar-jack mixture.)

1 additional cup shredded low-fat cheese (If you buy the two-cup package of cheese, you're covered.)

Preheat the oven to 400°.

Cook pasta according to package directions. Drain. Mix with cheese sauce. (I like to make the pasta and the sauce at the same time so the stirring isn't so boring—I can stir the sauce for a while, give the pasta a stir, stir the sauce some more … yes, I have a short attention span).

Put half pasta mixture in a casserole or other deep baking dish. Top with ½ cup shredded cheese. Top with remaining pasta and remaining cheese.

Bake for 30 minutes or until cheese is melted. Serve with a big salad and a bowl of fruit. It's pure simplicity.

The Secret Is in the Sides

Lest you think I'm only interested in dessert and gooey casseroles, let me assure you that one of the best ways to make a good meal into a great meal is to be creative with side dishes. Round out your yummy meals with side dishes such as the following:

◆ A big, fresh, green salad filled with yummy raw vegetables and a delicious home-made dressing. Try this one:

Gluten-Free Salad Dressing

A go-anywhere oil-and-vinegar dressing.

1 cup extra virgin olive oil	**1 clove garlic, minced**
¹/₂ cup cider vinegar	**1 teaspoon dried herbs, crushed**
Juice from one fresh lemon or lime	
Dash of hot sauce or hot pepper flakes	**1 teaspoon salt**
	Freshly ground black pepper

Stir or shake together oil, vinegar, lemon juice, hot sauce, garlic, herbs, salt, and pepper, and serve immediately.

◆ The freshest seasonal vegetables chopped and sautéed quickly over high heat in canola oil flavored with a little sesame oil. Sprinkle with sesame seeds.

◆ Baked white potatoes topped with sour cream or plain yogurt and fresh chopped chives or salsa.

◆ Sweet potato fries. Cut sweet potatoes into strips; toss with canola oil and a little cinnamon-sugar or salt; and bake at 400° until tender and just starting to crisp, about 30 minutes.

◆ Homemade salsa or pico de gallo.

◆ Pretty pilaf. You can press a lot of different gluten-free grains into pilaf form. Try these:

Toss cooked rice, quinoa, or millet with chopped nuts and fresh herbs or some finely chopped tomatoes and onions. Press into an ice cream scoop or a ¹/₂ cup measure, and turn out onto plates for a classy side dish. Garnish with a parsley, cilantro, or mint leaf.

Fearless Eater

I love this recipe for super-simple Pico de Gallo. I eat this a lot, and I also like to mix it half-and-half with avocadoes for a chunky heavenly guacamole.

Pico de Gallo

2 tomatoes, cored, seeds squeezed out, chopped

½ white onion, peeled and chopped, then rinsed in a colander (makes it taste sweeter)

1 clove garlic, peeled and minced

1 fresh jalapeño, seeded and minced

½ cup fresh cilantro leaves, chopped

½ teaspoon kosher salt

Juice of one fresh lime

Combine all ingredients in a big bowl and serve with corn chips or on potatoes.

Now, we hope you're gotten some great ideas from this chapter and will enjoy inventing your own versions of these recipes. Gluten-free cooking is so much fun if you take it as a challenge and stretch your creativity. Who needs wheat? Not you! You're cooking gluten-free.

The Least You Need to Know

◆ If your pantry is well stocked with gluten-free ingredients, you'll always have what you need to cook delicious gluten-free meals.

◆ Baking with gluten-free flour is easier if you practice a few special techniques, like chilling the dough before baking, adding binders like applesauce, and not expecting your creations to taste *exactly* like baked goods made with wheat flour.

◆ Be creative with one-pot meals for easy gluten-free suppers.

◆ Side dishes add flair and flavor to your meals.

Chapter 14

A Week of Gluten-Free Menus

In This Chapter

◆ Foods to eat all week

◆ Your personal gluten-free shopping list

◆ Start making your own menus

You've learned about gluten-free products. And you've learned about gluten-free cooking. But how do you put it all together? Why, devise a gluten-free menu plan, of course! In this chapter, we'll give you seven healthy, delicious, gluten-free breakfasts, lunches, dinners, and snacks. Mix and match in whatever way you like, or feel free to adjust things according to your own preferences. We're here to serve.

For this chapter, we won't be including portion sizes because these would vary so much according to your individual needs. Some people with celiac disease have suffered such a nutritional deficiency that once they start healing, they may feel the need to eat a little more. Others may start gaining too much weight, once their bodies start to heal and take in more nutrients, and may need to eat a little less. We hope you won't feel frustrated that these pseudo-recipes don't give exact amounts. This is freestyle cooking—a little of this, a little of that. Just add what you think looks good. None of these meals are complicated.

But they do offer healthy, balanced nutrition. You can increase or decrease the actual calorie amount as well as ingredients according to your needs and tastes. Also see Chapter 17 for more information on healthy eating and finding *your* ideal weight on a gluten-free diet.

Beautiful Breakfasts

Start the day out right with gluten-free breakfasts like these. You might also want to add a glass of water with lemon or a cup of tea, herbal, green, or black, or coffee, decaf, regular, or the carob variety without actual coffee beans.

Breakfast #1

I find toast so very comforting. I don't know why, but I'm sure it has something to do with my mom (who has been known, now that she doesn't have to cook for her kids anymore, to eat nothing but toast for dinner). Toast is also quick and simple. I eat this breakfast often.

Good for You

If you choose soy, rice, or almond milk, Tricia says to be sure to choose varieties that are not only gluten-free but also fortified with calcium and vitamin D.

- Gluten-free bread (preferably whole-grain or enriched), toasted, spread with almond-butter or any other nut butter and jam or jelly. We like the all-fruit jams better than the kind loaded with sugar.

- Fresh pineapple chunks or any other fresh fruit you like.

- One percent, skim milk, or gluten-free soy, rice, or almond milk.

Breakfast #2

This yummy hot breakfast is perfect for dreary, rainy mornings or cold, snowy days. I like Bob's Red Mill Brown Rice Farina Creamy Rice Hot Cereal with gluten-free vanilla rice milk. Walnuts are a great addition to hot cereal, too, and are an excellent source of omega-3 fatty acids.

- Hot rice cereal with real maple syrup and a light sprinkling of chopped walnuts and raisins.

- One percent, skim, or gluten-free, calcium and vitamin-D-fortified soy, rice, or almond milk.

- Fresh strawberries.

Breakfast #3

For a heartier breakfast or for when you really crave some protein, try this one. You can spice it up by adding some chopped jalapenos or a dash of hot sauce. I've been known to throw in a few cubes of avocado, too, when I have it.

- Scrambled egg (or scrambled tofu) cooked with chopped green onions, diced tomatoes, and fresh cilantro. Or toss with your favorite salsa.

- Warm corn tortillas, preferably whole grain.

- Orange slices lightly dusted with cinnamon-sugar or calcium-fortified orange juice.

Breakfast #4

The gut-friendly bacteria in yogurt can help with digestive issues, and yogurt is full of calcium and protein, too.

- Plain low-fat or nonfat yogurt (regular or soy), topped with fresh berries or snipped dried apricots, a few sunflower seeds or sliced almonds, and a drizzle of honey or real maple syrup. Or try chocolate syrup, if you want to have this for dessert—so much healthier than an ice cream sundae!

- Half a grapefruit or grapefruit juice.

Breakfast #5

Sometimes you just want some pancakes or waffles, and fortunately, you can have them if you always have some gluten-free pancake and waffle mix around. I put lots of different things in pancakes, according to what I have around the house: fresh or frozen berries, sliced bananas, walnuts and raisins, or chocolate chips.

You also can get some delicious gluten-free premade waffles. Tricia's favorite breakfast is a whole-grain gluten-free waffle topped with all natural peanut butter, frozen blueberries, and a little real maple syrup. Heat the blueberries and the syrup in the microwave first. Yum! Now you know what professional nutritionists eat for breakfast.

- Gluten-free pancakes. Use gluten-free pancake mix, make the blueberry pancakes in Chapter 13, or try waffles, filled or topped with fresh berries and/or peanut or other nut butter, just like Tricia does!

- Real maple syrup.

- 1 percent or skim milk, or gluten-free, calcium- and vitamin D-fortified soy, rice, or almond milk.

Breakfast #6

If you love to use your blender, breakfast smoothies are fun to make. Many people like to add yogurt or milk to their smoothies for added protein and calcium. I think the taste is cleaner and fresher with just the fruit and a banana for creaminess, so make it whatever way appeals to you. If the banana or the berries are frozen, this smoothie will be thick and icy like a milkshake. This will get you started in your smoothie experimentation:

- Berry smoothie. Combine one banana (fresh or frozen) *or* $1/2$ cup low-fat yogurt or milk, one cup fresh or frozen berries (strawberries, raspberries, blueberries, or whatever you happen to have), and $1/2$ cup orange or pineapple juice. If it's not sweet enough for you, add one tablespoon real maple syrup or honey. For extra spice, add a dash of cinnamon or a sprinkle of nutmeg.

- Gluten-free whole grain crackers with your favorite nut butter or a little bit of apple or fig butter.

Breakfast #7

This is one of my oldest son's absolute favorite breakfasts. Years ago, we saw something like this described in a magazine and changed it to suit ourselves. Yummy!

◆ Banana delight. Spread peanut, almond, or soy butter all over the surface of a peeled banana. Drizzle a little honey over the peanut butter, and roll the banana in any whole or enriched ready-to-eat gluten-free cereal. We like the Nature's Path crispy rice or Perky O's. Or try Enjoy Life Granola. Eat with a fork.

◆ One percent or skim milk, or gluten-free, calcium- and vitamin D-fortified soy, rice, or almond milk.

Fearless Eater

Recently, I've noticed that the price on almond butter has more than doubled in my local store. I've heard the grower price for organic almonds has skyrocketed in the last few years, and maybe that's why. In any case, I don't eat almond butter as much as I used to. When I already spend extra money on gluten-free products, that $12 jar of almond butter can seem pretty extreme. Natural peanut butter works for me, but if you can't eat peanuts, you might consider soy butter.

Luscious Lunches

Lunch should give you enough well-rounded nutrition to get you through the afternoon but not be heavy or high-fat, or you'll start nodding off around 3 P.M. We recommend serving lunch with sparkling water served with a lemon or lime slice or a glass of herbal tea, hot or iced. Are you ready to "do lunch"? Let's go for it!

Lunch #1

Isn't tuna salad the quintessential lunch? I know a lot of people who think so. Try this healthy version.

◆ Tuna salad crunch. Mix water-packed (not oil-packed) light tuna (not albacore, which is high in mercury), drained, with a tiny bit of mayonnaise and minced celery, shredded carrot, and pickle relish. Or mix it with salsa. Serve on top of gluten-free (plain) rice cakes.

◆ Mixed green salad with gluten-free dressing.

Lunch #2

I like this lunch whenever I have leftover rice.

◆ Quick stir-fry. In a nonstick pan with a drizzle of olive oil over medium-high heat, sauté onion, garlic, bok choy, snow peas, carrots, or whatever vegetables you have, along with an egg or any leftover beef, chicken, fish, or tofu. Season with gluten-free tamari or gluten-free soy sauce. Serve over brown rice.

◆ Apple or any other fresh fruit, if you need something sweet to top off your meal.

Lunch #3

Bring this to work, and everyone will want to know what you're eating. Give them a taste, and they'll want the recipe.

◆ Cold quinoa salad. Combine cooked quinoa, canned kidney beans or white beans (drained and rinsed), chopped green onions, shredded carrots, the juice of one fresh lemon, finely chopped raw spinach, and just a drizzle of extra virgin olive oil. Season with salt and pepper to taste.

◆ Orange or tangerine slices. Eat them alone or better yet, mix them into the above salad.

Good for You

To stay within daily recommendations for cholesterol, Tricia advises limiting egg yolk consumption to no more than one per day or less if you eat other cholesterol-rich foods. Adding more egg whites is just fine, though, because the white part has no cholesterol but lots of protein.

Lunch #4

I love egg salad. It is my favorite lunchtime comfort food. I think I've mentioned before that I like to eat it with tortilla chips. I also like this curried version:

◆ Curried egg salad. Chop hardboiled eggs. Mix one yolk with the whites from several eggs— my dogs like to gobble up the other yolks, and I figure it's okay for them *once in a while*. Mix a small amount of mayonnaise, gluten-free brown mustard, minced celery, chopped walnuts, and just about $1/2$ teaspoon curry powder into the eggs. Roll mixture up in big leaves of romaine lettuce.

◆ Tomato salad. Toss chopped tomatoes with a drizzle of extra virgin olive oil, balsamic vinegar, and fresh chopped basil.

Lunch #5

This is my favorite lunch when I'm craving Mexican food:

◆ Fajitas. Warm up corn tortillas, and fill with cooked fish, chicken, beef, or black beans, a little low-fat cheese, and cooked onions and green pepper strips. Top with salsa and just a smidgen of sour cream.

◆ Mixed green salad with gluten-free dressing.

Lunch #6

A lot of people, and not just vegetarians, love vegetarian chili. It's low in fat, high in flavor, and quick to make if you pick up a good gluten-free canned variety like Amy's Medium Chili with Vegetables. Or make your own.

◆ Vegetarian chili. Sauté onions and garlic in a little olive oil. Add pinto or black beans, drained and rinsed if canned, a can of crushed tomatoes, and some chili powder. You can also add corn, carrots, green peppers, hot peppers, or other veggies—the more, the better! Add water if it gets too thick. Simmer until heated through.

◆ Brown rice or corn tortilla wedges. This is optional, although some people like to serve chili over brown rice or dip toasted tortilla wedges into their chili.

Lunch #7

Potatoes taste great with salmon. Try this delicious salad for lunch:

◆ Potato salmon salad. Cut a potato into cubes and boil for 15 minutes, or cut leftover potato into cubes. Sauté a salmon filet with a little onion, green pepper, and garlic. Mix with the cubed potato, and serve over salad greens, drizzled with fresh lime juice and a little olive oil.

◆ Orange or tangerine slices.

Delightful Dinners

I don't know about you, but I look forward to dinner all day long. In fact, I keep hinting to everybody else in the family that I wouldn't mind at all just spending all day planning dinner, as a career. They just roll their eyes at me because they know perfectly well I'm never going to stop writing books. But, I digress! Dinner is your chance to sit down with the people you love and enjoy delicious food. What could be better? Here are some ideas to help inspire *you*.

Fearless Eater

Sometimes, I'll have a glass of wine with dinner, or gluten-free beer if dinner's on the spicy side. Often, I'll just have some juice mixed with club soda in a wine glass. Try it—it feels elegant, and it's good for you.

Dinner #1

This hearty home-cooked meal will make everybody feel cozy. I often cook this for my family but make a few tofu cutlets on the side for me. I marinate them the same way, but in a different bowl, for any interested GF-Vegetarians out there.

◆ Herbed chicken. Marinate chicken breasts or tofu slices in a mixture of olive oil, fresh lemon juice, minced garlic, oregano, and thyme, in a shallow covered pan or Ziploc bag, for at least three minutes. Broil or grill.

◆ Sweet potato fries. Peel sweet potatoes, cut into fry shapes, spray with gluten-free nonstick cooking spray or olive oil, sprinkle with sea salt or brown sugar, and bake at 400° for about 30 minutes.

◆ Tossed green salad with gluten-free dressing.

◆ Fresh cherries or frozen if out of season.

Dinner #2

When I was in Paris, I loved to order the *omelette de fromage*. It was fun to say—much more fun than saying "cheese omelette." It's fun to eat, too.

◆ *Omelette de fromage.* Beat 2 eggs (or 1 egg and two egg whites) lightly with a little milk or water, and pour into a pan. Top with a little crumbled goat cheese and a sprinkle of fresh or dried tarragon. Flip one side over the filling, and cook until the egg isn't runny anymore. Garnish with chopped green onions or fresh chives.

◆ Thick tomato slices with fresh basil.

◆ White grape juice mixed with club soda.

◆ Fresh strawberries tossed with just a sprinkle of balsamic vinegar.

Good for You _____

Just because you can't eat wheat, barley, and rye doesn't mean you shouldn't be getting your whole grains. To help ensure adequate fiber, iron, and B vitamin intake, it is very important that you consume the recommended amount of grain foods each day. According to the government's Dietary Guidelines for Americans, that means three or more ounces of whole-grain products per day out of a total of six ounces recommended grain products (for someone consuming 2,000 calories a day). The rest of the recommended grains should come from enriched or whole-grain products.

Dinner #3

At least once a week, we have our own version of a Mexican restaurant at home. This kind of food pleases kids and adults alike.

◆ Tostadas. Toast corn tortillas, preferably whole-grain, in the oven until crisp; then let everyone top his or her own according to personal preference. I put out the following in little bowls: refried beans, chopped meat, black beans, corn, shredded low-fat cheese, sour cream, red salsa, green salsa, pico de gallo (see recipe in Chapter 13), and guacamole. (I usually put refried beans, guacamole, and pico de gallo or green salsa on mine, but Ben and the kids are all about the ground beef, pork, or chicken.)

◆ Corn tossed with chopped red and green bell peppers.

◆ Homemade vanilla pudding. Scald $2^1/_2$ cups 1 percent or skim milk over medium heat. In a separate bowl, combine $^1/_4$ cup cornstarch, $^1/_2$ cup brown sugar, and a dash of salt. Stir in an additional $^1/_2$ cup milk and 1 teaspoon vanilla extract into the cornstarch mix until it turns into a paste. Add this to hot milk, stirring constantly until it gets thick and smooth. I keep pressing the paste against the side of the pan with a wooden spoon to help dissolve it. Cook for about five minutes. Cool slightly and serve. You can also add sliced bananas right before serving. Or add $^1/_4$ cup cocoa powder and $^1/_2$ teaspoon cinnamon to the cornstarch and brown sugar for Mexican-inspired chocolate pudding.

> **Good for You** _____
>
> Tricia advises sticking with low-fat milk, yogurt, and cheese, but advises caution when it comes to using low-fat and nonfat sour cream and mayonnaise and also nonfat cheese. She says that these products often contain fillers and gums to mimic the mouthfeel of fat. By contrast, low-fat milk, yogurt, and cheese are made simply by taking out fat. So go ahead and enjoy *small* amounts of real sour cream and mayonnaise, when appropriate. Just don't overdo it.

Dinner #4

Kabobs are fun for the grill, but they work great in the broiler as well. They also are good for families with lots of different dietary needs because everybody can have just the things they like.

◆ Kebobs. On individual skewers, thread cubes of steak, chicken, fish, or tofu, alternating with chunks of onion, green pepper, red pepper, tomato, mushrooms, artichoke hearts, and summer squash. Brush lightly with olive oil, and grill or broil until meat is done and veggies are tender.

◆ Potato salad. Mix cubed cooked white, yellow, or red potatoes and chopped vegetables, like celery, carrots, and red bell peppers, and toss with your favorite gluten-free salad dressing.

◆ Fresh mango with lime juice and coconut flakes. Or blend mango chunks, fresh lime juice, and pineapple juice with crushed ice for a frosty dessert drink.

Dinner #5

Often people who go gluten-free think they have to forgo pasta until they discover the gluten-free kind. This gluten-free spaghetti with meatballs brings all those good feelings back again.

◆ Spaghetti and meatballs. Cook and drain rice or quinoa spaghetti or any other gluten-free pasta, preferably whole-grain or enriched, according to package directions. Sauté chopped onion, garlic, and mushrooms. Add tomato sauce and tomato paste, or your favorite gluten-free jarred pasta sauce, and dried oregano. Simmer until heated through. Serve with plain, extra-lean ground beef or ground turkey rolled into balls and cooked. You don't need bread crumbs, but use crumbled gluten-free bread and egg if you want to mimic your favorite meatball recipe. Or serve this without the meatballs.

Fearless Eater

When everybody else is eating meatballs, I like to make "meat"balls out of 100 percent soy TVP (textured vegetable protein) soaked in warm water until it resembles ground meat (follow package instructions for soaking—it only takes a few minutes). It's easy to shape and tastes pretty similar once it's in the sauce, especially if you mix in a little salt, pepper, and dried sage before shaping into balls. Bob's Red Mill makes 100 percent soy TVP.

◆ Garlic bread. Roast whole garlic bulbs in the oven for about an hour at 350°. Squeeze out the paste on gluten-free bread, drizzle with olive oil, and broil for just a minute or two until golden.

◆ Tossed green salad with gluten-free dressing.

◆ Low-fat frozen yogurt, gluten-free of course, topped with your favorite berries.

Good for You

If you don't have the patience to roast a bulb of garlic, just mince the garlic and spread it on the bread or on gluten-free crackers for a quick-and-easy, Italian-inspired accompaniment to pasta.

Dinner #6

Sometimes, I just want a big salad for dinner. On those days when you want to keep it light, throw all your fresh veggies into a big bowl and spike them with leftover meat, hardboiled eggs, beans, tofu, and/or nuts. Top with gluten-free dressing. Here's one version my family likes:

◆ Broccoli dinner salad. Combine lots of chopped broccoli, chopped red bell peppers, cooked green peas, chopped hardboiled eggs, chopped celery, and a few chopped walnuts in a big bowl. (Optional: add a little cubed turkey breast.) Whisk together olive oil, fresh lemon juice, a little gluten-free brown mustard, and some minced garlic. Add red pepper flakes if you like it spicy. Pour over salad, and toss to coat.

◆ Favorite fruit salad. As long as you're mixing it up, mix together whatever fresh fruit you have in the house, too. For a tropical twist, try pineapple cubes, orange slices, banana slices, and a little flaked coconut. Or for an orchard blend, mix cubed apples, peaches, plums, and green and red grapes.

Dinner #7

Soup's on! Soup is so easy and delicious and comforting, we barely eat anything else at home during the winter. It's also flexible so, once again, you can make it anything you want it to be. I often make mine in the slow cooker.

◆ Sensational soup. In a soup pot or slow cooker, combine chopped onion, minced garlic, finely chopped bitter greens, like collard greens or kale, mushrooms, a can of crushed tomatoes, some chicken or vegetable broth (gluten-free), brown rice or quinoa (it will cook in the broth) and a little bit of any leftover meat, poultry, fish, beans, or tofu you have in the refrigerator. Simmer for one hour, or let it cook in the slow cooker all day.

◆ Home-baked bread. Use one of the delicious gluten-free bread mixes, like Pamela's Wheat Free Bread Mix or one of Bob's Red Mill whole-grain gluten-free bread mixes, and make some bread, either in the bread machine or by hand, to go with your soup. Go ahead; it's therapeutic, and it's *so good* warm out of the oven.

◆ Peach crisp. Put sliced peaches sprinkled with fresh lemon juice in a pie pan. In a small bowl, combine $1/2$ cup rice flour, $1/4$ cup brown sugar, one tablespoon chopped almonds or walnuts (optional), one teaspoon cinnamon, and a dash of salt. Mix in one tablespoon melted butter. Sprinkle mixture over peaches, and bake at 350° until peaches are tender, about 40 minutes. Serve with a dollop of low-fat vanilla yogurt.

Happy Snacking

When you can't quite wait until your next meal, have a healthy but delicious snack. Fruit is always a good choice, but sometimes you might want something a little more substantial. Try these options on for size:

◆ Frozen berries, orange slices, and pineapple juice mixed in the blender with or without a dollop of yogurt for a quick fruity smoothie

◆ Gluten-free energy bar, such as a Lärabar

◆ Gluten-free whole-grain or enriched cold cereal with low-fat or skim milk

◆ Pineapple chunks or grapes in fat-free or low-fat yogurt

- Whole-grain gluten-free crackers with peanut, almond, or soy butter

- Figs smeared with goat cheese

- Baby carrots dipped in gluten-free hummus

Your Weekly Shopping List

This shopping list contains everything you need if you were to eat all the meals listed in the above sections. Make a photocopy, and take it with you! It looks long, but you probably already have a lot of this stuff. You can also cut the ingredients from any of the meals in this chapter you don't intend to make.

Good for You _____

Calcium is very important for sufficient nutrition. To help ensure adequate calcium intake, you should be consuming three one-cup equivalents of milk or milk alternatives each day. That includes low-fat milk, low-fat yogurt, low-fat cheese, calcium-prepared tofu, calcium-fortified orange juice, calcium-fortified soy milk ... or even cups and cups of cooked collard greens!

Depending on where you live, you may not be able to find gluten-free bread, pasta, pancake mix, breakfast cereal, and other gluten-free products in your local grocery store, although an increasing number of "regular" grocery stores have gluten-free sections or sections specifically for people with allergies, which might contain gluten-free products. A better bet for the best selection is your natural food store or food co-op.

Produce

Avocados

Baby carrots

Bananas

Basil, fresh

Berries, fresh or frozen

Bok choy

Broccoli

Butter

Carrots

Celery

Cherries, fresh

Cilantro, fresh

Corn, fresh, frozen, or canned when out of season

Garlic

Grapefruit

Grapes, red or green

Green bell peppers

Green onions

Mango

Mushrooms

Lemons, fresh

Limes, fresh

Onions

Oranges or tangerines

Peaches

Pineapple, fresh

Plums

Potatoes, white or yellow

Spinach, raw

Red bell peppers

Romaine lettuce

Salad greens

Snow Peas

Strawberries, fresh and frozen

Summer squash

Sunflower seeds

Sweet potatoes

Tomatoes

Meat/Dairy

Cheese, low-fat

Chicken

Eggs, large

Goat cheese

Ground beef or ground turkey

Meat: steak, pork, chicken, etc.

Milk: 1 percent, skim, or gluten-free fortified soy, rice, or almond milk

Salmon filets

Sour cream

Tofu, prepared with calcium

Turkey

Yogurt, frozen, low-fat, or nonfat

Yogurt, plain or flavored, nonfat, or low-fat

Pantry Items/Miscellaneous

Almond butter, peanut butter, and/or soy butter

Almonds, sliced

Apple or fig butter

Artichoke hearts, in a jar or can

Balsamic vinegar

Black beans

Bread mix, gluten-free, whole-grain or enriched

Bread, packaged, gluten-free, whole-grain or enriched

Broth, chicken and/or vegetable, gluten-free

Brown mustard, gluten-free

Brown rice

Canned crushed tomatoes

Chili, vegetarian, canned, gluten-free

Cold cereal, gluten-free, whole-grain or enriched

Corn tortillas, whole-grain

Energy/snack bars, gluten-free

Extra virgin olive oil

Figs, dried or fresh

Honey

Hummus, gluten-free

Jam or jelly, preferably the all-fruit variety

Maple syrup, real

Mayonnaise

Pancake mix, gluten-free

Pasta sauce, in a can or jar, gluten-free

Pickle relish

Pineapple juice

Plums

Quinoa

Raisins

Refried beans

Rice cakes, plain, gluten-free

Rice cereal, hot

Salad dressing, gluten-free

Salmon filets

Salsa, red and green

Sea salt

Spaghetti or other pasta, gluten-free, whole-grain or enriched

Tamari or soy sauce, gluten-free

Tuna, light, canned

Vanilla extract

Walnuts

Spice Aisle/Baking Aisle

Brown sugar

Chili powder

Cinnamon

Cocoa powder

Coconut flakes

Cornstarch

Curry powder

Oregano, dried

Red pepper flakes

Tarragon, fresh or dried

Thyme, dried

Vanilla extract

Beverages

Club soda

Coffee, regular or decaf

Grapefruit juice

Orange juice, calcium-fortified

Tea, herbal, green, black, etc.

White grape juice

Meal-Planning Secrets

We hope that looking at these menus has given you some ideas for your own meal plans. Meal planning is so much easier if you actually plan the meals *before* the actual day you eat them. If you can set aside one day a week to sit down, write out the weekly meals, and make a shopping list, you'll be way ahead of the game ... and you'll never end up starving with nothing in the house to eat or staring into the open refrigerator wondering what you can possibly cook for dinner.

So many websites have gluten-free recipes that you could spend hours just browsing them and dreaming about what you could eat next (we list some of these in Appendix B). When you run out of ideas, just type "gluten-free recipes" in your browser and hit "search."

Also, keep a journal of the meals you eat and how you like them. You'll never be left wondering, "What was that great dinner I made last month that the kids just loved? What the heck *was* that?"

Finally, just keep trying. Don't get frustrated. Many, many former noncooks have transformed into competent and even highly skilled gluten-free chefs in their own homes, out of necessity, and eventually out of the sheer love of preparing food at home that actually tastes good. Good luck! And *bon appétit*.

The Least You Need to Know

- There are plenty of gluten-free food choices to cover breakfast, lunch, dinner, and snacks.

- Plan your meals ahead, and make a complete shopping list so you always have something to make and eat.

- Be patient as you explore this new universe of food; you may have to try a recipe several times or experiment with different meal choices to get it just right for you, but the final product will be worth it.

Part

Out and About: Gluten-Free and Loving It!

If you think the grocery store is confusing, just wait until you try to explain gluten to a waitress who doesn't know what you're talking about! In Part 5, we explore the restaurant scene, from formal to casual, take-out to fast food. We even help you find food on the road and guide you in smart snacking. We also look at some of the health implications of a gluten-free diet. Will you lose weight? Gain weight? Will you get the right nutrients? We give you guidelines so you can be sure to attain your healthy best.

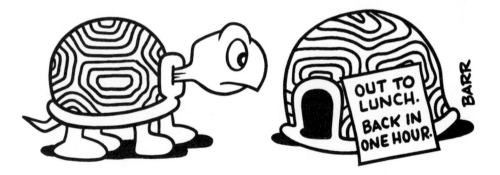

Restaurant Scoreboard

In This Chapter

◆ Choose your restaurant wisely

◆ Translating your needs to the waitstaff

◆ Gluten-free fast food

◆ A list of gluten-free-friendly restaurants

I admit it: I love to cook, but sometimes, I just don't *feel* like cooking. I'm guessing you don't either—at least, not every single night for the rest of your life. Going out to eat is *fun*. It's *social*. It *gets you out in the world*. You don't want to do that every night either, of course—that would get expensive, not to mention fattening and pretty limiting, as far as gluten-free choices. However, once in a while, it's really nice to go out to a restaurant and have somebody else do the cooking—and the cleaning up—for a change.

But eating gluten-free in a restaurant can be very challenging, too. Some establishments are incredibly willing to work with you, but others don't have a clue what you are talking about when you mention the "g" word. Sometimes, the chef knows what contains gluten and what doesn't, but the waiter or waitress doesn't and, consequently, makes false assumptions, giving you the wrong information. You end up "getting glutened," which really destroys the whole enjoyable aspect of eating out. What's a gluten-free restaurant-goer to do?

It would be great if we could print out a comprehensive list of every restaurant with all the gluten-free items they offer. But the fact is, menus change constantly, and recipes for foods on restaurant menus change, too, as different ingredients become available or sometimes just according to the whim of the chef. Whisk a little flour into that soup to thicken it up? Why not? Someone who doesn't care about gluten wouldn't mind or think twice about it, but that kind of spur-of-the-moment creative cooking can spell disaster for you and your gut.

But you *can* eat out successfully and still stay gluten-free if you find the right places to go and know the right way to talk to the waitstaff or, if necessary, the chef him- or herself. This chapter will help enable you to do this.

Choosing Your Restaurant

The first trick for successful gluten-free eating while eating out is to choose a restaurant where you can actually *be* successful. Frankly, some restaurants have virtually nothing gluten-free on the menu, but many others have plenty of choices or will accommodate you by changing dishes to make them gluten-free.

In general, although there are certainly exceptions, nicer, high-end restaurants are usually eager to accommodate the special needs of diners. We dropped over a hundred bucks at a steakhouse recently, but the food was great; the service was superb; and the waitress and chef were very careful to be certain every item on my plate was entirely gluten-free. The waitress even offered to put the bread basket at the farthest possible point on the table away from me, but next to Ben, who ate it all.

But sometimes, mistakes happen. Sometimes, servers aren't well informed. Sometimes, part of an entrée will be gluten-free, but another part won't, and the server won't realize this. Fish can be dusted with flour; sauce might be thickened with flour or flavored with wheat-containing soy sauce; soups often contain gluten ingredients; dressings might contain wheat, and sometimes, servers don't really know what gluten *is*, so they wouldn't know how to advise you.

As celiac disease and gluten-free eating become increasingly common or at least well known, more and more restaurants are educating all their employees about what gluten is and what foods contain it, but occasionally, you may encounter it by accident. Tricia says she can almost always find something to eat in a restaurant, with the possible exception of Italian restaurants. She tends to frequent nicer restaurants where she knows she can eat something.

When in doubt, Tricia suggests fresh broiled fish with lemon or melted butter (stress no breadcrumbs or flour!), a preparation that lets the real flavor of the fish come through. The fresher and better the fish, the less we want to drown the flavor in fatty sauce. Sides could be broiled or baked potatoes with a little salt, a dab of butter, or a splash of olive oil and whatever fresh herbs they have on hand. Or try fresh hot rice. Steamed vegetables have a crisp, bright flavor if they aren't overcooked, or have a salad filled with whatever produce is in season. A lot of restaurants have some version of this on the menu. Vinaigrette dressing is usually a safe bet, too. When all else fails (or when you feel like something a little more indulgent now and then), you can usually find nachos on the menu. Just make sure the restaurant uses natural cheese and not cheese sauce. That's what I usually do at a local place my family likes to go.

Fearless Eater
Recently, Tricia went to an Italian restaurant in Laguna Beach (Pomodoro) where the rest of her family wanted to go. She was looking over the menu thinking she would have to stick with the tomato, mozzarella, basil salad (good choice, by the way, and usually available) when right there on the menu she read that gluten-free noodles were available. For the first time in years, Tricia was able to order a pasta dish right off the menu!

Also, many chain restaurants are particularly committed to providing allergy information and have special (if changing) allergy menus, as well as gluten-free menus. Remember, many restaurant staff will talk to you about gluten as if it's an allergy—which, although not exactly accurate, is really fine as long as they are helping you to avoid gluten. Many of these restaurants post their menus on their websites, updating them frequently. You might have to call others, but do so ahead of time and find out what you can order so you know you aren't wasting a trip. The last section of this chapter will provide you with a list of some of the major chain restaurants that are usually gluten-free-friendly.

Other things to consider:

◆ Call ahead to find out if the restaurant can accommodate you. If they don't seem to know what you are talking about or don't think they have anything, don't go there.

◆ If your server doesn't speak English very well, explaining your dietary restrictions may be difficult. Consider this when choosing a restaurant—although also remember that ethnic restaurants are likely to offer the widest variety of gluten-free options.

◆ Don't go out to eat at the busiest times. Servers can get stressed out and will be less willing to listen to a long explanation or make accommodations when they have a lot of tables and need to hurry. If you go out to eat earlier or later in the evening than the typical dinner rush, you will probably get a more responsive server. Call the restaurant to find out what times are less busy.

Translating Gluten-Speak to Your Waiter or Waitress

You walk into the restaurant. The hostess shows you to your table. You sit down. The waiter hands you a menu. Now what?

Before you order, explain right away to your server that you can get very ill if you eat anything made with gluten, including flour, wheat, rye, barley, oats, or malt flavoring. Don't go on and on. Be succinct. Ask the server for help in recommending a dish, or ask whether the chef can prepare something appropriate for you.

Fearless Eater

When ordering in a restaurant, don't assume anything—servers might think "wheat flour" means "whole-wheat flour" and often don't know what other ingredients typically contain gluten. It's best to get your recommendation directly from the chef, but even after you've received a recommendation, confirm that the dish you are ordering has no flour, wheat, rye, barley, oats, or malt flavoring and that it isn't made with sauces containing flour or with flavorings like soy sauce or beer. It's better to be safe than sorry! And remember, it's just fine to be a high-maintenance diner as long as you tip well.

Ordering off the Fast-Food Menu

We don't recommend eating fast food very often—it's usually pretty high in fat and low in nutrition. However, many fast-food restaurants have taken strides to offer healthier choices, and once in a while, you will probably find yourself faced with a drive-through run or a quick stop-in for lunch.

When you order fast food, you don't have a server. You order all by yourself, which can make things easier, in a way. However, it can be tough to find fast food without gluten. So many things are breaded or fried in a fryer that fries things that are breaded, like French fries fried with breaded chicken nuggets. Remember these tips for ordering gluten-free in fast-food restaurants:

- ◆ Ask if they publish a gluten-free menu or a brochure with nutritional information. Many fast-food restaurants do—for a few of them, see the list at the end of this chapter.

- ◆ Order a sandwich—hold the bun! These days, nobody will think twice about this kind of order; they'll just think you're on the Atkins diet. Many restaurants now also offer lettuce wraps for the low-carb set. And the gluten-free set benefits, too!

- ◆ When in doubt, stick with a salad if it comes without the croutons already on the salad. Read salad dressing labels carefully.

Gluten-Free-Friendly Restaurants

Obviously, we can't list every restaurant in the world in this book, and we can't even list every restaurant with a gluten-free menu on its website. The following are some popular chain restaurants in many cities that specifically address gluten on their websites with menus and ordering advice. We apologize in advance to any restaurant we have left off this list—these are the ones we know about. We certainly hope you will find more!

Good for You _____

If you want more local or customized information about which restaurants are gluten-free-friendly, check out the www.glutenfreerestaurants.org website of the Gluten-Free Restaurant Awareness Program, which lists many restaurants around the country. Search by restaurant, city, state, country, or cuisine. Also check out Triumph Dining at www.triumphdining.com. They publish a comprehensive restaurant guide. These resources will give you more information about individual locations.

Of course, remember that local restaurants can be great places to eat. You support your local economy and they get to know you and your special needs, so whenever you can, eat locally! Otherwise, here are some options for you to consider:

- ◆ **Bennigans.** They don't have a gluten-free menu, but they say on their website that they will do their best to accommodate special dietary requirements. Call first. The "Talk to Us" link on the website includes their statement about accommodating special dietary requirements. Go here to find out more: www. bennigans.com.

◆ **Bonefish Grill.** A great seafood restaurant chain for gluten-free eating in many different states (mostly in the eastern half of the country so far with lots in Florida where the restaurant originated), this restaurant has a gluten-free menu on its website, with individual items clearly labeled with a big "**GF.**" Go to www. bonefishgrill.com, and click on "Tasty Bites," then click on "Download our Gluten-Free Menu." Sweet!

◆ **Burger King.** You can find a Burger King just about anywhere in the world, and this fast-food chain's website makes it easy to find things you can eat. Many, many of their menu items contain wheat, but a few don't, and the website tells you not only what items have wheat but also which are cooked in fryers with other ingredients containing allergens. As of today (but check to be sure), they cook their fries in a dedicated fryer, so those are gluten-free. It's a very informative website, and that's pretty handy, even if you find out you can only order a salad and some fries. Go to www.bk.com and type "Gluten Free" in the box at the top of the screen. Click on "Go."

Good for You _____

Many gluten-free eaters bring their own dressing, soy sauce, or even gluten-free pasta into restaurants, and we've never encountered a restaurant who minded. If you bring your own pasta, ask if the chef will prepare it for you in a separate pot, and mention that gluten-free pasta cooks quickly and will get mushy if it sits in hot water too long. When you find a chef willing to do this, you know you've found a gluten-free-friendly restaurant. If you frequent a place you know is sympathetic and knowledgeable about your dietary needs, they will get to know you, and then you'll get even better treatment. Be sure to tip well! It can't hurt.

◆ **Carraba's Italian Grill.** Known in gluten-free circles for their gluten-free friendliness, Carraba's has many locations around the country and a link on their website to their gluten-free menu. Go to www.carrabbas.com/menu.asp, and click on the Gluten-Free Menu download link. Not only does it tell you the gluten-free items on the menu, but it also tells you exactly which special requests to make for which menu items, such as "Request no pasta added" next to the soup and "Request to be made without grill baste" next to the grilled items.

◆ **Chick-fil-A.** For fast-food chicken, Chick-fil-A offers gluten-free chargrilled options (order without the bun of course) to their breaded filets, plus lots of other gluten-free items. Find out what's gluten-free at Chick-fil-A *right now* at www.chickfila.com/gluten.asp. The list is refreshingly long.

◆ **Chili's.** This family-friendly restaurant has a gluten-free menu on its website, although they also have a disclaimer that says that because of the risk of cross-contamination in a busy kitchen, they "are unable to guarantee that any menu entrée below can be prepared or are wheat/gluten-free." They also suggest not ordering anything fried because different foods are all fried in the same fryers. At least they are honest! Even so, they do list "Suggested Menu Options for wheat/gluten allergies," so if you decide to go to Chili's anyway, you'll have some ideas. Ask when you get there anyway, however, just to confirm that what you are ordering really is gluten-free or that the chef can take special precautions to make it so. For the menu options list, go to www.chilis.com, click on "Menu," click on "Allergen Info," and then click on "Wheat and Gluten Allergen Information."

◆ **Chipotle.** This Mexican restaurant lets you choose exactly what you want, and they make it while you watch. So you can order tacos filled with whatever you want and can see exactly what is touching the flour tortillas. I ate here the other day while I was in Indianapolis and tried one of their burrito bowls—burrito ingredients without the tortilla. It was really yummy and very economical. Check them out at www.chipotle.com to find a Chipotle near you.

◆ **Claim Jumper Restaurants.** Nice restaurants with bars located in many states, Claim Jumper Restaurants have a gluten-free menu on the website. But they also warn that the establishment is not gluten-free and that the menu items on the gluten-free menu have been modified to be gluten-free, so you have to specify this desire to the server. Still, they offer many choices, perfect when you are in the mood for a nice gourmet salad or a good piece of grilled salmon. Check out the gluten-free menu at www.claimjumper.com. Enter the site, click on "menus," click on "dietary concerns," and then click on "gluten-free."

◆ **Cold Stone Creamery.** Are you in the mood for ice cream? Cold Stone Creamery's website tells you which flavors *do* contain gluten, and they also warn that while they clean the stone often, they can't guarantee your ice cream won't be cross-contaminated with an allergen. However, many of their flavors do not contain wheat or gluten, so if you ask them to clean the stone really really well first, you may decide to go for it. Care for dark chocolate peppermint, anyone? For their allergen list, go here: http://www.coldstonecreamery.com/assets/pdf/nutrition/Allergen_Chart_11_06_06.pdf.

◆ **Culver's.** Another fast-food favorite, Culver's advertises frozen custard shakes and butter burgers. Not exactly low-calorie fare, but they do have a gluten-free menu on the website via a cool nutrition calculator that lets you click on any menu item.

It shows you all the ingredients and nutritional information for that item, plus allergy alerts. Then you can take off elements (like the bun) and re-calculate to see how the nutritional information changes. However, the allergy alerts stay the same, so you'll have to figure out if removing the bun, for example, removes the gluten. Go to www.culvers.com and click on "Nutrition Choice Calculator."

Good for You

Desserts can be tough for the gluten-free diner, but most restaurants have ice cream or sorbet on the menu (usually not alone but served with other wheat-laden desserts). When Tricia feels like dessert, she asks for just the sorbet or ice cream and has never been told no. But if you go this route, stress no cookies on the side. You don't want them to ruin a perfectly good dish of ice cream by chunking a couple of gluten-y cookies in the middle.

◆ **Dairy Queen.** Dairy Queen has a gluten-free product list on its website, although they ask you to reconfirm the gluten content of any menu item with your local Dairy Queen. They list the flavors, bars, slushes, coffee drinks, and toppings without gluten. Go to www.dairyqueen.com, click on "Menus and nutrition," click on "Special Dietary Needs," and then click on "Gluten-Free Products."

◆ **First Watch.** This "daytime café" serves breakfast, brunch, and lunch only and has a thorough gluten-free menu on its website. They tell you what you can order and what to specify, such as "no muffin" or "no granola" to make the order gluten-free. They also add that occasionally, products may be substituted or product ingredients could change, so always order with caution—sensible advice for *any* restaurant-dining gluten-free eater. Look here: www.firstwatch.com/pages/menus_glutenfree.html.

◆ **Legal Seafood.** This upscale seafood chain, based in Massachusetts, has locations up and down the East Coast. They even cater weddings. Every location has a gluten-free menu, which includes children's items, and the company takes allergy and other dietary concerns very seriously. Go here and they'll know exactly what you need. Check them out at www.legalseafoods.com. Their menu isn't on the website, but this is one place you won't have to worry about.

◆ **McDonalds.** McDonalds has complete nutritional and allergy information for each menu item on its website. Go here, http://app.mcdonalds.com/bagamcmeal; then "Add Items" to your virtual "bag," and click on "Get the Nutrition Facts," then on "More Details."

◆ **Outback Steakhouse.** One of the best gluten-free-friendly choices, the ubiquitous Outback Steakhouse makes it particularly easy to order gluten-free. They've got lots of items on their gluten-free menu, and it's easy to find. Just go to www.outbacksteakhouse.com, click on "Our Menu," and then click on "Gluten Free Menu" link toward the bottom of the page. It's very thorough with specific ordering information for each item, like "BBQ sauce is GF" or "Avoid the Cabernet sauce."

> **Fearless Eater**
>
> Tricia's husband is from California, and when they visited recently, he wanted to go to In-N-Out Burger. Tricia had heard they had a "secret menu" with a special "Protein Style" burger that comes without the bun. She hadn't ordered a fast-food burger in years, but she tried it … just because she could. Check it out at www.in-n-out.com/secretmenu. asp. Next time you go, you'll be in the know.

◆ **P.F. Chang's.** Another gluten-free-friendly choice, this Chinese restaurant chain, found in many states, has a detailed gluten-free menu on its website. Go here: www.pfchangs.com/cuisine/menu/glutenIntolerantMenu.pdf. As of this printing, they even have a menu item called "Singapore Street Noodles" containing "shrimp, chicken, and rice noodles stir-fried in gluten-free sauce." You won't find that at a restaurant very often … gluten-free noodles! That alone could be worth a trip.

◆ **Subway.** I stopped here the other day with the whole family on the way home from spring break and was happy to find that many of their salads are gluten-free. On its website, their gluten-free menu also tells you exactly which sandwich fillings, sauces, etc. are gluten-free. Go to www.subway.com, and click on the "Menu/Nutrition" drop-down menu, select "Nutrition," and then click on "Food Allergies Information."

◆ **Taco Bell.** Taco Bell seems like it might have a lot of options, but it doesn't. There are a few, though. Go to www.tacobell.com, click on "Nutrition Guide," and then click on "Food Allergens and Sensitivities. Taco Bell lists both wheat and gluten, marking ingredients that could potentially bother someone with a sensitivity. This list will tell you what they are.

◆ **Wendy's.** Wendy's continually updates their gluten-free menu online and actually has quite a few gluten-free choices. Find out what they are by going to www.wendys.com, clicking on "Nutrition," then clicking on "Menu Items Without Gluten." Simple! I really like the taco salad. Also, as of today, the chocolate and new vanilla frosties are gluten-free, in case you were wondering. Always check first, though, to be sure this hasn't changed.

The Least You Should Know

- Ordering gluten-free in a restaurant can be challenging. Call ahead to be sure the restaurant can accommodate you.

- If the server isn't sure what you are talking about, ask if you can speak with the chef.

- Check to see if restaurants have gluten-free menus online.

- Always check for updated gluten-free information, and never assume anything you order is gluten-free. Always ask! Recipes in restaurants can change.

Take Out (or Take Along)

In This Chapter

- ◆ Reasons for always having gluten-free foods with you
- ◆ Make it a potluck
- ◆ Great gluten-free take-along ideas
- ◆ Gluten-free lunches from home
- ◆ Foods to send off with gluten-free kids

You're out and about, tooling around town in your car, and hunger strikes. When you visit a friend, she brings out a plate of cookies. You get invited to a wedding, and everything on the buffet is glutted with gluten. What do you do?

You could swing through the drive-through (see Chapter 15), but you know that's not very healthy. You could decline the cookies and watch hungrily as your friend eats or feel guilty that she has to abstain to make you feel better. You could just stare at the wedding cake and feel bummed out. Or … you could be prepared.

When you eat gluten-free, you will often find yourself out in the world and hungry, with nothing to eat. And that's when you'll be awfully tempted to cheat even though you know you'll regret it. Don't do that to your body!

Instead, carry gluten-free foods with you at all times. People with asthma carry inhalers, so why shouldn't you carry some gluten-free snacks in your purse or in your car?

When it comes to gluten-free eating, planning is everything. If you are always ready to be confronted with gluten, you'll never end up starving with no options. This chapter will help prepare you.

Stock Your Purse, Briefcase, or Glove Compartment

Always carry gluten-free snacks in your purse, briefcase, or car, for every-day running around town. You never know when you might get caught in traffic or running errands and suddenly get hungry. Some great choices for on-the-run noshing:

- Energy bars like Lärabars or gluten-free Genisoy bars
- Rice cakes (gluten-free varieties, of course)
- Microwave popcorn
- Small Ziploc bags filled with nuts or seeds
- Gluten-free crackers or breadsticks and packets of nut butter (These handy packets are good for use on the rice cakes, too—you can also find packets of jelly and cream cheese. One source: www.scoutgear.com/funfood.html.)
- Fruit (a classic)

Brown Bag-It

Why spend money at a restaurant every day? Lunch is healthier, and cheaper, if you bring your own. In a lunch box, brown bag, or a fancy cooler, you'll be satisfied with these gluten-free goodies:

- Veggies and a little low-fat cheese wrapped in warmed corn or rice tortillas and then wrapped in plastic so the wrap holds its shape.
- Sandwich on gluten-free bread. Try gourmet versions like apple slices with almond butter, turkey slices with pear, or hummus with greens and a splash of vinegar.
- Lentils cooked with onions, garlic, and carrots, over brown rice and tossed with vinaigrette dressing.
- Gluten-free soup. Just heat and eat. (Your office has a microwave, right?)

Life Is a Potluck

Potluck or not, all social events could be potential disaster for gluten-free eaters—or potential great times. However, you must be prepared. Whenever you get invited to any social event that will involve food, you need to do one of three things:

1. Talk to the host or hostess about your dietary restrictions, and offer to bring your own food so nobody else has to worry about you.

2. Eat before you go so you aren't hungry and won't have to worry what might be served, unless it's a dinner party, in which not eating would be rude.

3. Decline the invitation.

Now that last choice isn't any fun, so let's go with the first two options, instead.

BYOGFF

That stands for Bring Your Own Gluten-Free Food, in case you weren't sure. Who doesn't appreciate someone bringing food to a social event? Whenever you get invited to anything, ask if you can bring a dish. Explain that you have a special diet but don't want anyone to feel they have to change their plans, so you are more than happy to bring something to share … something that conforms to your needs, but that you hope others can enjoy, too.

Your hostess might say no and insist on cooking something you can eat. If so, great! Explain your needs. But offering to help out by bringing your own food makes life easier on everyone—especially you. Plus, you won't be stuck nibbling on carrot sticks while everybody else feasts on spaghetti and garlic bread.

Fearless Eater

Ben and I have a lot of parties, some of them more formal than others. For dinner parties, there are several things we really dislike. First, when people don't RSVP. We can't plan the amount of all the courses very well if we don't know how many will attend. Second, when people don't show up on time. Dinner parties, especially with themes, must be carefully timed with the cooking. Finally, when people don't make their dietary requirements clear ahead of time. We recently had a fancy multi-course Italian dinner, and over half the attendees, unbeknownst to us, said they couldn't or wouldn't eat at least half the courses, for various dietary reasons. We would have been happy to accommodate those needs if only we had known ahead of time!

Don't be afraid to tell your hostess what you can and can't eat, and certainly don't decline just because you are afraid to be a bother. RSVP, show up on time, and work with the hostess *before* the party to plan out what you can and can't eat and what parts you can bring for yourself.

For ideas about what you could bring to a party, see Chapters 12 and 13. Tricia's friends all know to put out rice crackers, partly because she always serves them at her house and people love them, but if your friends haven't discovered how delicious they are, enlighten them by bringing some along.

Or consider any of the following:

- A big salad with lots of fresh veggies, some nuts or seeds, or some chickpeas or black beans topped with a gluten-free dressing.
- Gluten-free whole-grain pasta, cooked and tossed with your favorite sauce.
- Sandwiches, all done up in your favorite gluten-free bread and filling. Peanut butter and jelly, anyone? Paté? Spinach salad?
- Gluten-free crackers with goat cheese, nut butter, and other healthy spreads, or canapés made on toasted squares of gluten-free bread.
- Soup, filled with all your favorite gluten-free veggies.

Spoil Your Appetite

Yes, we know, your mother always told you *not* to spoil your appetite before dinner, but if you eat before you go out with friends or attend a social event, you won't have to worry about what they're serving. "No thanks, I'm really full," is a fine response to a plate of gluten-y h'ors d'oeuvres. Plus, if you're not starving, you can concentrate more on socializing.

Formal Functions

Whether it's a wedding, a business dinner, or whatever, sometimes you just can't turn the event into a potluck. It wouldn't be appropriate to haul your slow cooker of gluten-free stew to your cousin's wedding reception.

If the event is catered or held at a restaurant, it is important to call the restaurant and discuss your dietary needs ahead of time. Don't bother your boss or the bride about it. You may prefer to be served the same food with slight modifications to make it gluten-free—this prevents long explanations about your dietary restrictions when everyone is supposed to be courting the client or complimenting the happy couple. However, sometimes this isn't possible, and your meal may look very different from theirs. However, you decide how much you want to discuss your gluten-free diet; you can always just say it's for medical reasons and change the subject.

If the affair is serve-yourself with a buffet table or h'ors d'oevre tray, there is almost always cheese and raw vegetables. It is perfectly fine to eat the cheese without the cracker. If you miss the cracker, then bring some from home. Also look for fruit, sliced meat, sandwich fixings without the bread, and, of course, salad as long as it isn't doused in croutons.

Travel Savvy

Traveling can be difficult enough without food concerns. Add in the uncertainty of not knowing what will be available to eat, and a trip can become very difficult unless you are prepared.

Tricia says she always travels, whether by plane, train, or automobile, with a gluten-free cache that includes rice cakes, nonperishable peanut butter in a plastic tub (yes, the unhealthy kind, believe it or not!), Genisoy bars and Lärabars, dried fruit and nut mixture (she's partial to pumpkin seeds and papaya), and gluten-free cookies. Tricia loves Enjoy Life Foods brand chocolate chip cookies. She finds that breakfast and snacks are the most difficult times for her to find gluten-free foods away from home. With her gluten-free cache, she has her own breakfast and snacks, no matter what might be offered elsewhere.

When I last hit the road, I brought my own cache of gluten-free snacks, and I never once had to go browse the gas station for something to eat. With a cup of coffee and a Pamela's ginger cookie, I was quite satisfied.

Particularly when traveling by plane since you obviously can't stop at that gas station, always plan ahead to carry on some gluten-free food. Whatever is small but nutrient-dense makes an efficient travel snack. Think nuts, dried fruit, and energy bars. If you've got a long flight ahead, and the flight includes a meal, call ahead to request a gluten-free meal. Most airlines can accommodate this, if you make arrangements ahead of time.

However, those snack boxes you can buy on the planes all contain some gluten—at least, all the ones we've seen. Plus, many people with celiac disease do not trust the airlines to put together gluten-free meals—sometimes they come with items that clearly are not gluten-free. Some airlines are better than others, but even if you do order gluten-free meals on your plane ride across the country or across the world, we strongly suggest bringing your own gluten-free food on board, just in case.

Prepare Family Members

You might not be the only one in your family who has to eat gluten-free. Many of us have gluten-free kids, and like it or not, they are often out of sight.

You wouldn't send your child to school without her gluten-free lunch, so why send her to a friend's house without a gluten-free snack? Kids aren't always good about sticking to the rules, and it's easy to get hungry and accept a graham cracker here, a goldfish cracker there, and an Oreo cookie then and again.

When your child goes to a friend's house, tell the parents about his or her dietary restrictions. Most parents are pretty savvy about allergies today because of the increase in peanut allergies—they will understand. And nip on-the-sly snacking in the bud by making sure your gluten-free kids always have snacks, too. Give them a special lunch-box or purse just for holding their gluten-free snacks. You'll probably like some of these snacks, too:

◆ Low-fat cheese sticks

◆ Gluten-free cracker or rice cake and peanut butter "sandwiches"

◆ Hardboiled egg

◆ Apple and/or pear slices with peanut butter for dipping

◆ Grapes (better than candy!)

◆ The occasional gluten-free cookie (if they're going to eat cookies, make sure they are gluten-free so your kids aren't getting their cookies on the sly)

◆ Hummus and baby carrots

◆ Healthy trail mix: nuts, seeds, raisins, dried cherries, coconut, chocolate chips, or whatever else your child likes

◆ Homemade gluten-free cereal bars (follow the directions for your favorite cereal bar recipe, substituting gluten-free cereal for regular)

For more information on kids and celiac disease, look at the list of books in Appendix B.

So you see, eating gluten-free away from home isn't so bad after all, as long as you have everything you need with you. You might even find a great vintage lunchbox for the purpose—who says kids have to have all the fun? Of course, what you carry your gluten-free food *in* is less important than just having it with you.

Do that, and, to misquote from *Gone with the Wind* (and just know I'm saying this in my very best Scarlett O'Hara accent), "*As God is your witness, you'll never be hungry again!*"

Good for You _____

If kids are provided a snack at school (ubiquitous in preschools and kindergartens and common for the first half of grade school, too), provide the school with a cache of gluten-free snacks. These days, your child probably won't be the only one with a dietary restriction.

The Least You Need to Know

◆ Always offer to bring your own gluten-free food to social events, so you aren't stuck with nothing to eat.

◆ Work with your hostess to coordinate your needs with the needs of her party.

◆ Eat before social events so you don't have to worry about eating *at* social events.

◆ Bring your own lunch—it's healthier and cheaper.

◆ Make sure your gluten-free kids always have snacks with them, too, so they won't be tempted to eat the snack foods their friends are eating.

Get Ready to Get Healthy, Gluten-Free!

In This Chapter

◆ Nutritional challenges of gluten-free eating

◆ Results of changing your diet

◆ Finding your ideal weight, gluten-free

◆ Making the most of every bite

Are you underweight and achy? Overweight and bloated? Tired all the time? Feeling better now but gaining weight at an alarming rate?

Eating gluten-free in a healthful way is a little more complicated than just eating gluten-free. You've almost certainly gone gluten-free because eating gluten was making you sick, but now that your diet is more in line with your body's needs, are you sure you're getting all the nutrition you need?

Perhaps you fit the classic profile of the person with celiac disease who is underweight with chronic digestive issues. Or maybe you don't fit that classic profile, and would really like to get back *down* to a healthier weight. You might also have other health issues to deal with, either temporarily until you heal, such as lactose intolerance, or permanently, such as diabetes, or other auto-immune diseases that often go hand in hand with celiac disease. Whatever your situation, you'll be happy to know that your food choices can do more than stop hurting you. They can actually help you.

The Gluten-Free Diet: What's Your Version?

Just because you can't eat gluten doesn't mean you can dine only on cheeseburgers without the bun and gluten-free cookies and expect to be healthy or feel good. Where's the fiber? How's your calorie count? How much fat did you eat today? Did you get enough calcium, folate, and iron? If you aren't thinking about these questions, then your gluten-free diet may not be a particularly healthy one. And if you are eating too many calories, too much fat, and too little fiber and nutrients, your diet certainly isn't going to help you lose those extra pounds you may have found creeping around your middle since your body started to heal and absorb nutrients more efficiently.

But eating gluten-free *and* nutritiously can be challenging for you as a gluten-free eater because you feel so darned *deprived* that you just want to find something, anything gluten-free. Plus, you might feel that after all you've been through, you *deserve* the gluten-free cookies or the cheeseburger or the giant platter of nachos or French fries or whatever it is you've chosen to make up for the gluten-filled goodies you miss.

Luckily for you, your co-author, Tricia, is a registered dietitian, who knows exactly what you should be eating, and in this chapter, she's here to tell us. So let's start with Tricia's favorite subject: whole grains.

Healthy Whole Grains

There are gluten-free grains, and there are gluten-free *whole* grains. The word *whole* makes a big difference. When you first go gluten-free, you can be so excited to find a bread mix or a box of cookies without gluten that you'll gobble up anything (I know I did.) Then, you start to feel it—either your waistline starts to widen, you get constipated, or you just don't feel so great.

Whole grains contain, as you might guess, the whole grain, including the germ and the bran. They have many more nutrients than processed refined grains, and more fiber, too. If you're feeling constipated, you may not be getting enough whole grains, and even if you *aren't* feeling constipated, you may not be getting enough fiber.

According to the Dietary Guidelines for Americans, jointly published in 2005 by the United States Department of Health and Human Services and the United States Department of Agriculture, at least half the grains you eat should be whole grains. The rest should at least be enriched grains. Otherwise, those grains are really just calorie-laden starches and not much use to your body beyond some quick energy. When you need to eat gluten-free, every bite counts, so why waste any of your "bites" on non-nutritious starch when you could have nutrient-packed whole grains?

Some gluten-free whole grains, like brown rice, are easy to find in your local grocery store. But others are harder to find. Look in Chapter 9 and Appendix B for lists of some excellent producers of gluten-free whole and enriched grain products. And we've also pointed you toward one source we know of for each grain below. Many of these grains are also widely available in natural foods stores. Try to include these gluten-free whole grains in your diet:

- **Brown rice.** This staple is much more nutritious than its white counterpart and should be available in grocery stores.

- **Buckwheat.** Look for whole buckwheat groats, kasha (roasted buckwheat groats), or 100 percent buckwheat flour. Buckwheat works well in pancakes and as a side dish. Find it at www.thebirkettmills.com.

- **Amaranth.** Look for amaranth grain and flour. Amaranth works well in baked goods. Find it at www.nuworldfoods.com.

- **Sorghum.** Sometimes called milo, this is a staple grain in Africa. Sorghum flour is often used in gluten-free baked goods. Find it at www.twinvalleymills.com.

- **Whole oats.** Use guaranteed gluten-free varieties only. Find them at www. pure-oats.com or www.glutenfreeoats.com.

- **Teff.** This tiny grain is commonly used to make bread in Ethiopia. Look for teff grain and teff flour. Teff works well in baked goods and as a breakfast cereal. Find it at www.teffco.com.

- **Corn, including popcorn.** Look for whole-grain cornmeal in the ingredients list. Corn products are widely available in grocery stores.

♦ **Millet.** This grain has a bland flavor but tastes great in soup or other flavorful dishes needing a little extra bulk. Find it at Bob's Red Mill brand: www. bobsredmill.com.

♦ **Quinoa.** This food has a mild grainlike flavor and excellent nutritional profile. Quinoa works well as a side dish. Find it at www.quinoa.com and www.quinoa. net.

♦ **Wild rice.** This grain is native to the United States and Canada. It has a nutty, chewy flavor and is widely available in grocery stores and natural food stores. It works well added to rice mixtures.

Fiber Facts

Fiber comes from the part of plants your body doesn't digest, so it moves everything along, keeping your digestive system working properly. Too much can give you gas (especially if you aren't used to it), but most people only get about half as much fiber as they should. The recommended amount is between 21 and 38 grams per day, depending on your age and gender. Fiber helps reduce your cholesterol level and is associated with a decreased risk of certain cancers, especially colon cancer. It also helps keep you regular.

Whole grains are an excellent source of fiber. So are fruits, vegetables, and legumes. In fact, legumes are such a great source of fiber and nutrients that I try to include them in my diet every day. After your gut has started to heal and you can digest more roughage, eating beans regularly helps your body adjust to them. Eventually, they may not give you any gas at all. Some of them are also milled into flour, like soy flour and garbanzo bean flour. Some legume varieties we enjoy:

♦ Adzuki beans

♦ Black soy beans

♦ Black turtle beans

♦ Black-eyed peas

♦ Chickpeas/garbanzo beans

♦ Kidney beans

♦ Great northern beans

- ◆ Green lentils

- ◆ Red lentils

- ◆ Mung beans

- ◆ Pinto beans

- ◆ Soybeans

- ◆ Navy beans

- ◆ Red beans

- ◆ Split peas, green and yellow

Good for You

Flax seed. Whole or ground up into meal, flax seed is rich in Omega-3 fatty acids (similar to fish) and fiber. Many grocery stores and most health food stores carry flax seed.

The packaged foods you eat should also be whole grain and high-fiber whenever possible. Look for whole grain gluten-free breakfast cereals, breads, and pasta with at least 2.5 grams of fiber per serving … because ironically, the more bulk you have in your food, the less bulk you could have around your middle. Fiber helps fill you up so you might be less likely to overeat.

Folate, B-Vitamins, and Iron: Are You Getting Enough?

Unlike most refined wheat-based foods, most refined gluten-free breads, flours, and pastas, as well as breakfast cereals, are not enriched with B vitamins and iron. So people with celiac disease may have to work a bit harder to get adequate amounts of these nutrients, which is one reason why it is so important to choose whole-grain or enriched grain products when eating gluten-free.

Folate is a particularly important B-vitamin for women capable of becoming pregnant. It is recommended that these women consume 400 micrograms of synthetic folic acid from enriched food or supplements in addition to food sources of folate, such as broccoli, collards, orange juice, asparagus, garbanzo beans, and lentils. Folate supplementation is one reason why enriched gluten-free grain foods are important.

Whole and enriched gluten-free grain products are also a good source of other B-vitamins, including thiamin, riboflavin, and niacin, as well as the mineral iron. Consuming adequate amounts of iron is especially important for people with celiac disease, especially because some people with celiac disease may suffer from iron-deficiency anemia. Companies that enrich their gluten-free products include Ener-G Foods, Enjoy Life Foods, Perky's, Heartland's Finest, Kinnikinnick, Pastariso and Pastato brand pasta, and Glutino. For contact information, see Appendix B.

Fruits and Veggies

If you want something sweet, how about having a juicy-sweet piece of fruit? Tricia says whole grains, vegetables, and fruits should be the center and primary focus of your meals. These plant-based foods contain vitamins, minerals, fiber, and carbohydrates for energy. Choosing plenty of fruits and vegetables every day is incredibly important for regaining and maintaining your health. Variety is paramount—eat with the seasons; choose what's fresh; and stock up on frozen options, too.

If you eat about 2,000 calories every day, you should be eating about 2¹/₂ cups of vegetables (one cup of vegetables is equivalent to one cup raw or cooked or two cups leafy greens) and about two cups of fruit (one cup of fruit equals one cup raw fruit, one cup fruit juice, or ¹/₂ cup dried fruit). Every week, choose from the five subgroups of vegetables, including those that are dark green, orange, and starchy.

Good for You _____

For more specific information about how much of each food group to include every day, check out the U.S. government's food pyramid at www.mypyramid.gov, as well as the Dietary Guidelines for Americans at www.health.gov/DietaryGuidelines.

Low-Fat Protein

If you can't eat wheat, you probably get plenty of protein because it's one of the things you *can* eat without worrying too much about it, as long as it isn't breaded. However, if you are concerned about your waistline, your heart health, or your cholesterol levels, you should choose your protein sources wisely.

How much protein you need each day depends on your age, gender, and activity level. A person requiring 2,000 calories a day requires five and a half one-ounce equivalents from the "meat and bean group" each day. One-ounce equivalents include:

- One ounce lean meat or poultry
- One ounce fish
- ¹/₄ cup or two ounces of calcium-prepared tofu (plain)
- One ounce cooked gluten-free tempeh
- ¹/₄ cup of cooked legumes

- One egg

- One tablespoon nut butter

Calcium

Many people don't get enough calcium, even though all you need are three one-cup equivalents from the milk group, which includes the following:

- One cup milk, low-fat or nonfat

- One cup low-fat yogurt

- One and $\frac{1}{2}$ ounces low-fat cheese

- One cup soy, rice, or almond milk, gluten-free, calcium-fortified

- One cup calcium-fortified orange juice

- Calcium-prepared tofu, amount should contain approximately 300 milligrams of calcium

Also, some vegetables are good sources of calcium, such as collards (one cup) and rhubarb (one cup). However, if you are a vegan who eats no animal products and not using calcium-fortified products, it can be difficult to take in adequate calcium from food. Talk to your physician and/or dietitian about taking a calcium supplement.

As a result of celiac disease, some people develop a secondary form of lactose intolerance. These individuals can't break down the milk sugar lactose because they lack the enzyme lactase. This usually resolves as the intestine heals. However, even with lactose intolerance, you can still consume milk-based products. Lactaid brand milk has zero lactose, and hard cheeses are low in lactose. Also, yogurt with active live cultures is generally well tolerated.

Weight Management

As your body starts to heal and absorb nutrients again and as you slowly figure out how many foods you really can eat, you may start to gain weight. That's okay if you need to gain weight, but if you don't or are already a few pounds over, you may need to make some adjustments.

Your doctor may have tips for you about the best ways to achieve your ideal weight, and, of course, you should follow your doctor's advice. But nutritionists know a thing or two, too, and we just happen to have one here at your disposal. Aren't you lucky?

First off, Tricia doesn't believe in diets. They work at first, but when you go off the diet (if you are like most), you regain the weight. (I certainly know what that's like!) She believes in making permanent, lifelong changes in eating habits. Base your meals on whole grains, vegetables, fruits, beans, nuts, seeds, fish, chicken, lean meat, and low-fat milk products or milk alternatives.

If you've made these changes and are still overweight, look more closely at some of your eating habits. Ask yourself some questions:

- Are you drinking too much sugary soda? Soda has a lot of calories with zero nutritional payoff. Consider phasing out your soda habit.

- Do you use high-fat condiments such as butter, margarine, mayonnaise, and salad dressings on a regular basis? Consider cutting down on these.

- Do you choose full-fat dairy products? Consider switching to low-fat milk, cheese, and yogurt.

- Do you regularly consume high-fat, high-sugar desserts and sweets like ice cream, gluten-free cakes, cookies, quick breads, etc.? That could explain an excessive calorie intake. Consider saving these treats for special occasions.

- Are you exercising less than you should? Shoot for about 30 to 45 minutes of exercise on most days. Your body will thank you. For more information on exercise, see the website www.hsph.harvard.edu/nutritionsource/exercise.htm.

Most people will answer "yes" to at least one of these questions, but if you already follow these basic principles and still want more help with your diet, Tricia recommends checking out www.mypyramid.gov, an interactive website that helps you determine how much you should be consuming from each of the food groups based on your individual needs.

The Least You Need to Know

- Eating gluten-free isn't necessarily enough to regain your good health; you also must make smart choices.

- Whenever possible, choose whole-grain products over refined and enriched over nonenriched.

◆ Eat plenty of fruits and vegetables; choose lean protein sources over fattier ones; and opt for low-fat over full-fat dairy products.

◆ Follow Tricia's tips for sensible weight loss to feel healthier and look fabulous.

Glossary

amaranth   A nutritious gluten-free grain.

arrowroot   A gluten-free starch used as a thickener.

barley   A grain containing protein similar to gluten, often used to make malt flavoring and to brew beer. People with celiac disease must not eat barley.

besan   A name for flour made from chickpeas.

bran   The fiber-rich, outer layer of a cereal grain.

buckwheat   A nutritious gluten-free grain.

bulgur   A form of whole wheat. Bulgur contains gluten.

cassava   A gluten-free starch. May also be referred to as manioc.

celiac disease   A genetic, autoimmune disease in which the body reacts to the proteins in wheat, rye, and barley (commonly called gluten) by damaging the intestinal *villi*—tiny hairlike protrusions in the small intestine that help absorb nutrients, resulting in problems absorbing nutrients.

celiac sprue   Another name for celiac disease.

couscous   A form of wheat. Couscous contains gluten.

cross-contamination   The term for a gluten-free food getting gluten on it by touching another food or gluten-contaminated surface.

dermatitis herpetiformis   The skin form of celiac disease; the disease manifests as a rash or hives rather than, or in addition to, other symptoms.

Dietary Guidelines for Americans   A document jointly published every five years since 1980 by the Department of Health and Human Services and the United States Department of Agriculture, to provide advice about good dietary habits. Find out more at www.health.gov/DietaryGuidelines.

disaccharide   A group of two units of sugar joined together that can be broken down into single units of sugar (monosaccharides) when hydrolyzed.

dinkle   Another name for spelt, a type of wheat. Dinkle contains gluten.

durum   A variety of wheat. Durum contains gluten.

einkorn   A variety of wheat. Einkorn contains gluten.

emmer   Another name for durum wheat. Emmer contains gluten.

enrichment   The process of adding vitamins and minerals to a food to increase its nutrient content.

FALCPA   An acronym for the Food Allergen Labeling and Consumer Protection Act, which took effect on January 1, 2006, requiring all FDA-regulated packaged food containing milk, eggs, fish, crustacean shellfish, peanuts, tree nuts, wheat, and soy to declare these common allergens clearly on the label.

FDA   *See* Food and Drug Administration.

flaxseed   A seed rich in omega-3 fatty acids. Flaxseed does not contain gluten.

Food and Drug Administration   Part of the United States Department of Health and Human Services, whose primary purpose is to regulate food and drug products to protect human health. Check out their website at www.fda.gov.

fu   Dried wheat gluten.

gliadin   Protein found in wheat gluten.

gluten   A protein found in wheat that gives dough its sticky, elastic quality. Some people have an autoimmune reaction to gluten and similar proteins in barley and rye. This condition is called celiac disease.

gluten intolerance   A nonspecific term that generally refers to an intolerance or sensitivity to the proteins in wheat, barley, and rye, either due to celiac disease or for some other reason.

gluten sensitivity   A nonspecific term that generally refers to an intolerance or sensitivity to the proteins in wheat, barley, and rye, either due to celiac disease or for some other reason.

gluten-sensitive enteropathy   Another name for celiac disease.

graham flour   A kind of wheat flour. Graham flour contains gluten.

hydrolysate   A compound formed by hydrolysis, which is the process of chemically breaking down a compound using water.

intestinal villi   Microscopic little fingers of tissue on the intestinal wall covered with even smaller little protrusions called microvilli. Villi greatly increase the intestine's surface area so the body can absorb digested nutrients more efficiently.

kamut   A variety of wheat. Kamut contains gluten.

legumes   A general term for beans, peas, lentils, peanuts, and similar plant foods. Legumes do not contain gluten.

lentils   A type of legume. Lentils do not contain gluten.

malt   Grain that has been soaked and sprouted. This process brings out the natural sugars in a grain. Under FDA regulations, the use of the term "malt" on the food label means it is made from barley. If malt is made from another grain, such as corn, the label must specify this, as in "corn malt." Malt contains gluten.

matza or matzo   Unleavened bread or its flour, made from wheat and contains gluten.

millet   A nutritious gluten-free grain.

milo   Another name for sorghum.

monosaccharide   A single unit of sugar, such as glucose that can't be broken down and occurs naturally or through hydrolyzing polysaccharides.

nontropical sprue   Another name for celiac disease.

polysaccharide   A long chain of monosaccharides joined together that can be broken down into smaller units.

quinoa   A nutritious gluten-free grain.

rye   A grain containing a protein similar to gluten. People with celiac disease must not consume rye.

seitan   Wheat gluten, often used in Asian or vegetarian "fake meat" products.

semolina   A form of coarsely ground wheat often used in pasta. Semolina contains gluten.

sorghum   A nutritious gluten-free grain.

spelt   A variety of wheat. Spelt contains gluten.

tapioca   A gluten-free starch often used for thickening.

taro   A gluten-free starch often used for thickening.

teff   A nutritious gluten-free grain.

tempeh   A fermented whole soybean product. Plain tempeh does not contain gluten, but many seasoned or flavored varieties do, so read labels carefully

tofu   Soybean curds made from coagulated soymilk. Plain tofu does not contain gluten, but many seasoned, flavored, baked, and smoked varieties do, so read labels carefully.

triticale   A grain that is a cross between wheat and rye. Triticale contains gluten.

villi   *See* intestinal villi.

wheat allergy   An allergic reaction specifically to wheat, rather than an autoimmune response to gluten. An acute condition, it comes on within about two hours after eating wheat and is most common in children. People with wheat allergies can't eat wheat, but can eat barley and rye.

whole grain   Grain processed along with the bran and germ that contains more vitamins, minerals, and fiber than refined grains.

Resources

Want to know more? Fortunately, plenty of great resources have cropped up all over the country (and the world) to help people eating gluten-free learn more, talk to others, buy the foods they can eat, and stay motivated. This appendix includes some of the resources we have found helpful.

National Celiac Disease Organizations

Celiac Sprue Association
P.O. Box 31700
Omaha, NE 68131-0700
Phone: 877-CSA-4-CSA (toll free)
Website: www.csaceliacs.org

Gluten Intolerance Group
31214 124th Ave., SE
Auburn, WA 98092-3667
Phone: 253-833-6655
Website: www.gluten.net

Celiac Disease Foundation
13251 Ventura Blvd. #1
Studio City, CA 91604
Phone: 818-990-2354
Website: www.celiac.org

Celiac Disease Medical Centers

Celiac Disease Center at Columbia University
161 Fort Washington Ave., Suite 645
New York, NY 10032
Phone: 212-305-5590
Website: www.celiacdiseasecenter.columbia.edu

University of Maryland Center for Celiac Research
20 Penn Street, Room S303B
Baltimore, MD 21201
Phone: 414-328-6749
Website: www.celiaccenter.org

Beth Israel Deaconness Medical Center
Nutrition Services, Rabb B06
330 Brookline, Avenue
Boston, MA 02215
Phone: 617-667-1272
Website: bidmc.harvard.edu/display.asp?node_id=5449

University of Chicago Celiac Disease Program
5841 S. Maryland Ave.
Chicago, IL 60637
Phone: 773-702-7593
Website: www.uchospitals.edu/specialties/celiac

Gluten-Free Cookbooks

Fenster, Carol. *Cooking Free: 200 Flavorful Recipes for People with Food Allergies and Multiple Sensitivities.* Avery, 2005.

Hagman, Bette. *The Gluten-Free Gourmet Cooks Comfort Foods: Creating Old Favorites with the New Flours.* New York: Owl Books, 2004.

Mallorca, Jacqueline. *The Wheat-Free Cook: Gluten-Free Recipes for Everyone.* New York: Morrow Cookbooks, 2007.

Roberts, Annalise G., and Peter H.R. Green. *Gluten-Free Baking Classics.* Evanston, IL: Surrey Books, 2006.

Sarros Connie. *Wheat-Free, Gluten-Free Cookbook for Kids and Busy Adults*. New York: McGraw-Hill, 2003.

Shepard, Jules E.D. *Nearly Normal Cooking for Gluten-Free Eating: A Fresh Approach to Cooking and Living Without Wheat or Gluten*. Seattle, WA: BookSurge Publishing, 2006.

Washburn, Donna, and Heather Butt. *The Best Gluten-Free Family Cookbook*. Toronto, ON, Canada: Robert Rose, 2005.

Gluten-Free Books and Magazines

Gluten-Free Living magazine. Website: www.glutenfreeliving.com

Bower, Sylvia Llewelyn, Mary Kay Sharrett, and Steve Plogsted. *Celiac Disease: A Guide to Living with Gluten Intolerance*. New York: Demos Medical Publishing, 2006.

Case, Shelley. *Gluten-Free Diet: A Comprehensive Resource Guide*. Regina, SK, Canada: Case Nutrition Consulting, 2006.

The Essential Gluten-Free Restaurant Guide, Second Edition. Arlington, VA: Triumph Dining, 2007.

Falini, Nancy Patin. *Gluten-Free Friends: An Activity Book for Kids*. Centennial, CO: Savory Palate, Inc, 2003.

Fine, Karen. *How I Eat Without Wheat*. Bloomington, IN: Authorhouse, 2007.

Green, Peter H.R., and Rory Jones. *Celiac Disease: A Hidden Epidemic*. New York: Collins, 2006.

Koeller, Kim, and Robert La France. *Let's Eat Out! Your Passport to Living Gluten and Allergen Free*. Chicago, IL: R & R Publishing, LLC, 2005.

Kruszka, Bonnie J., and Richard S. Cihlar. *Eating Gluten-Free with Emily: A Story for Children with Celiac Disease*. Bethesda, MD: Woodbine House, 2004.

London, Melissa, and Eric Glickman. *The GF Kid: A Celiac Disease Survival Guide*. Bethesda, MD: Woodbine House, 2005.

Peters, Jax Lowell. *The Gluten-Free Bible: The Thoroughly Indispensable Guide to Negotiating Life Without Wheat.* New York: Owl Books, 2005.

Ries, LynnRae. *Waiter, Is There Wheat in My Soup? The Official Guide to Dining Out, Shopping, and Traveling Gluten-Free and Allergen-Free.* Phoenix, AZ: What No Wheat Publishing, 2005.

Thompson, Tricia. *Celiac Disease Nutrition Guide.* American Dietetic Association, 2006.

Websites

American Dietetic Association: www.eatright.org

Celiac Sprue Association recipe page: www.csaceliacs.org/recipes.php

Celiac.com: A Celiac Disease & Gluten-Free Resource: www.celiac.com. Order gluten-free food, subscribe to the newsletter, or find recipes (type "recipes" in the search field). For their support group forum: www.glutenfreeforum.com.

Dietary Guidelines for Americans, 2005, available at: www.health.gov/DietaryGuidelines

Food Allergen Labeling and Consumer Protection Act, available at: www.cfsan.fda.gov/~dms/alrgact.html

Food and Drug Administration's proposed ruling on the use of the term gluten-free on food labels. Available at: www.cfsan.fda.gov/~lrd/fr070123.html

Gluten Free Beer Festival: www.glutenfreebeerfestival.com. Reviews and information for gluten-free beer lovers worldwide.

Gluten-Free Recipe Exchange: www.gluten.net/recipes

Harvard School of Public Health posting on exercise: www.hsph.harvard.edu/nutritionsource/Exercise.htm

Medications and Celiac Disease-Tips from a Pharmacist by Steven Plogsted: www.health.virginia.edu/internet/digestive-health/nutritionarticles/PlogstedArticle.Pdf

MyPyramid available at: www.mypyramid.gov

National Institutes of Health: www.nih.gov

National Institutes of Health Consensus Development Statement on Celiac Disease, available at: http://consensus.nih.gov/2004/2004CeliacDisease118html.htm

Questions and answers on the gluten-free labeling proposed rule available at: http://www.cfsan.fda.gov/~dms/glutqa.html

Recipe Zaar: This recipe site includes lots of gluten-free recipes: www.recipezaar.com/recipes/gluten-free

Sake World: www.sake-world.com

The Gluten Free Kitchen: gfkitchen.server101.com

Listservs and Online Support Groups

Yahoo! Silly Yaks online support group: health.groups.yahoo.com/group/SillyYaks

Yahoo! Vegetarian & Gluten-Free (VGF) group: groups.yahoo.com/group/vegetariangf

Yahoo! Gluten-Free Kitchen group: health.groups.yahoo.com/group/gluten-freekitchen

Yahoo! Gluten-Free Casein-Free Recipes (GFCFrecipes) group: health.groups.yahoo.com/group/GFCFrecipes

Yahoo! Food Allergy Kitchen group: groups.yahoo.com/group/FOODALLERGYKITCHEN

Yahoo! Vegan and Gluten Free group: groups.yahoo.com/group/Vegan-and-Gluten-Free

Celiac Listserve: www.enabling.org/ia/celiac

Manufacturers of Gluten-Free Foods

This list is not inclusive and not all of the foods made by all of these manufacturers are gluten free. Read labels carefully.

Amy's Kitchen (frozen meals and veggie burgers). Website: www.amyskitchen.com

Benedictine Sisters of Perpetual Adoration (low gluten alter breads). Website: http://benedictinesisters.org. Click on low gluten alter breads.

Bob's Red Mill (flour, hot cereal, and baking mixes, plus a good 100% soy TVP that's textured vegetable protein). Website: www.bobsredmill.com

Ener-G Foods (ready-made bread products, including sandwich-style, buns, rolls, and pizza crust, most gluten-free). Many products are enriched. Website: www.ener-g.com

Enjoy Life Foods (bagels, granola, cookies, snack bars). Many products are enriched. Website: www.enjoylifefoods.com

Gardenburger (so far, only one of their veggie burgers is gluten-free). Website: www. gardenburger.com

Genisoy (soy bars—but read the label because many of their bars are not gluten-free). Some gluten-free bars are fortified. Website: www.genisoy.com

Glutino (wide selection of products). Some products are enriched. Website: www. glutino.com

Health Valley (crackers, soups, but not all products are gluten-free). Website: www. healthvalley.com

Ian's Natural Foods (good kid food like fish sticks and chicken nuggets). Website: www.iansnaturalfoods.com

Kinnikinnick Foods (pre-baked bread, doughnuts, and many other choices). Some products are enriched. Website: www.kinnikinnick.com

Lärabar (dried-fruit-and-nut energy bars). Website: www.larabar.com

Lightlife (They make Tofu Pups, one of the few gluten-free vegetarian hot dogs. They also make gluten-free tempeh.) Website: www.lightlife.com/pups.html

Lundberg Family Farms (organic rice products of all kinds). Website: www.lundberg. com

Maple Grove Food and Beverage (pasta products, including some that are enriched). Website: www.maplegrovefoods.com

Nature's Path (cereals). Website: www.naturespath.com

Pamela's Products (cookies, biscotti, pancake and baking mixes). Website: www. pamelasproducts.com

Perky's Naturals (cereals). Many products are enriched. Website: www. perkysnaturalfoods.com

Sunshine Burgers (for gluten-free veggie burgers) Website: www.sunshineburger.com

Thai Kitchen (rice noodle instant soup, pad thai, noodle bowls) Website: www. thaikitchen.com

Tinkyada (pasta). Website: www.tinkyada.com

Van Harden's Pizza. Website: www.vanharden.com

Van's International Foods (waffles). Website: www.vansintl.com

Wild oats. Website: www.wildoats.com/U/department165/

Wildwood Organics (for gluten-free veggie burgers). Website: www.wildwoodfoods.com

Gluten-Free Grain Sources

Whole grains are such a great source of nutrition and fiber that we hope you'll explore the wonderful world of gluten-free whole grains. If you can't find very many interesting gluten-free grains in your local store, check out these sources (or check them out anyway—they might have better prices than your local store).

Amaranth: Nu World Amaranth (amaranth products. Website: www.nuworldfoods.com

Beans (not a grain but they make beans into flour, cereal, and pasta): Heartland's Finest (products made from beans, including enriched baking mix). Website: www.heartlandsfinest.com

Buckwheat: The Birkett Mills (buckwheat products). Website: www.thebirkettmills.com

Millet: Bob's Red Mill (wide variety of products including millet). Website: www.bobsredmill.com

Oats:

Chateau Cream Hill Estates (oats). Website: www.pure-oats.com

Gluten-Free Oats (oats). Website: www.glutenfreeoats.com

Quinoa: Northern Quinoa Corporation (wide variety of grains including quinoa). Website: www.quinoa.com

Rice: Lundberg Family Farms (organic rice products of all kinds). Website: www.lundberg.com

Sorghum: Twin Valley Mills (sorghum flour). Website: www.twinvalleymills.com

Teff: The Teff Company (teff grain and flour). Website: www.teffco.com

Gluten-Free Beer Sources

Anheuser-Busch Redbridge gluten-free beer. Website: www.redbridgebeer.com

Bard's Tale Dragon's Gold gluten-free beer. Website: www.bardsbeer.com

Lakefront Brewery New Grist gluten-free beer. Website: www.newgrist.com

Le Massagère gluten-free beer. Website: www.lesbieresnouvellefrance.com

O'Brien Premium Lager and Pale Ale. Website: www.gfbeer.com.au

Sutliff Hard Cider (not beer but a darned good stand-in). Website: www.sutliffcider.com

Gluten-Free Product Shopping Sites

Allergy Grocer. Website: www.allergygrocer.com

The Gluten-Free Mall (a wide variety of gluten-free products from many different manufacturers can be ordered from this website). Website: www.glutenfreemall.com

Shop Gluten Free (a wide variety of gluten-free products from many different manufacturers can be ordered from this website). Website: www.shopglutenfree.com

Whole Foods Market Gluten-Free Bakehouse. Website: www.wholefoodsmarket.com/products/bakery/gf_bakehouse.html

Gluten-Free Mini Cookbook

So you can't eat the same old foods. So what? You can eat new, exciting, amazing foods when you eat gluten-free. Plus, some of your old favorites might still be A-OK. In this mini cookbook, we give you lots of delicious recipes and ideas for what to eat, from soups and salads to main courses and desserts. And these recipes aren't grain-focused.

Instead, our recipes focus on fresh, seasonal ingredients that are not only delicious but also nutritionist-approved and oh-so-good-for-you. Plus, every single one is *easy* because if you are like us, you don't have hours to spend slaving over a hot stove.

So tie on your apron, and fire up your enthusiasm: it's time to eat well!

We intend all ingredients listed in the recipes in this appendix to be gluten-free, even if we don't say "gluten free" before the ingredient. So remember: always read the label! If a recipe calls for chicken broth or bacon or some kind of sauce or condiment or ice cream or whatever it is, always choose the gluten-free kind. (But we didn't really need to tell you that, right?)

Salads

I love a fresh, crisp salad on a hot summer day, but a salad *every* day is a great nutrient booster for anybody on a gluten-free diet. Salads make the best possible use of fresh seasonal ingredients and make you feel light and healthy, too. Plus, they are brimming with vitamins, minerals, and phytonutrients—what's not to love about a really good salad? Try these salad recipes, some perfect for summer, some warm and filling for colder weather, even a few sweet selections, for a fun and interesting way to get your daily dose of greens (and reds and oranges and yellows …).

Gluten-Free Chopped Salad

Fresh chopped vegetables blend with marinated flavors and cheese for a satisfying dinner salad.

16 large lettuce leaves (like romaine), shredded

1 tomato, seeds squeezed out and discarded, diced

2 radishes, cut into thin strips

6 scallions, finely chopped (white and green parts)

$\frac{1}{4}$ cup sunflower seeds or sliced almonds

16 olives, halved

1 4-ounce jar marinated artichoke hearts, cut into small chunks

4 ounces low-fat mozzarella cheese, cut into small cubes

4 ounces roasted red pepper strips (the marinated kind in a jar work just fine)

$\frac{1}{2}$ pound cooked shrimp, fresh tuna, shredded chicken, or garbanzo beans (optional)

Serves 4

1. Pile lettuce in the middle of a platter. Sprinkle tomatoes, radishes, scallions, and sunflower seeds or almonds over top.

2. Arrange olives, artichokes, cheese, pepper strips, and (optional) shrimp, tuna, chicken, or garbanzo beans around edges of salad. Lightly drizzle with about $\frac{1}{4}$ cup dressing (see following recipe), and serve extra dressing on the side.

Good for You

This simple chopped salad is meant to be messed with—don't take the listed ingredients too seriously. Substitute whatever looks best, freshest, and has traveled the shortest distance to get to your plate. If you choose to use the optional shrimp, fresh tuna, chicken, or garbanzo beans, this salad can be the centerpiece of the meal.

Dressing

Garlic, cheese, mustard, and optional hot sauce flavor this versatile dressing.

1 garlic clove, minced

1 shallot, minced

1 tablespoon grated Parmesan cheese

1 tablespoon gluten-free Dijon-style mustard

1/4 teaspoon kosher salt

Freshly ground black pepper

Dash of red pepper or Tabasco sauce (optional)

Juice from 1 fresh lemon

1/4 cup white wine vinegar or white wine

1/2 cup extra virgin olive oil

1. Combine garlic, shallot, Parmesan, mustard, salt, black pepper, red pepper, lemon juice, vinegar, and olive oil in a glass jar with a lid. Shake until combined.

Tomato Avocado Salad

Tomato, avocado, and lemon juice give this simple salad a salsa-esque flair.

2 tomatoes, halved, seeds squeezed out

2 ripe avocadoes, preferably Hass

1 tablespoon freshly squeezed lemon juice

$1/4$ teaspoon sea salt

2 tablespoons fresh cilantro, minced

2 scallions, minced

> *Serves 4*

1. Cut tomatoes into small bite-size wedges. Cut avocadoes in half, remove the pit, and cut slices into each half. To keep slices whole, remove them from skin carefully with a spoon. Combine tomatoes and avocado slices in a medium bowl or four separate salad bowls.

2. Drizzle tomato/avocado mixture with lemon juice, lightly sprinkle with sea salt, then top with cilantro and scallions. Serve immediately.

Good for You

This salad tastes delicious on its own or as a topping for fried eggs, a partner to tuna salad, or a side dish to a fresh plate of lightly dressed gluten-free pasta. Sometimes, this is all I have for lunch.

Green Pea Salad

Sweet green peas with savory turkey or cheese make this salad a filling meal.

Serves 4

2 cups cooked green peas, cold or hot

$^1/_2$ cup gluten-free deli turkey cut into matchsticks or $^1/_2$ cup shredded low-fat cheddar cheese (try both if you're really hungry or neither if you want a lighter dish)

$^1/_2$ cup red onion, finely chopped and rinsed in a colander

$^1/_2$ cup red bell pepper, finely chopped

$^1/_2$ cup yellow bell pepper, finely chopped

1 tablespoon extra virgin olive oil

Juice from 1 fresh lemon

1 teaspoon dried or 1 tablespoon fresh dill

$^1/_4$ teaspoon salt

Freshly ground black pepper

Combine peas, turkey or cheese, onion, red and yellow bell peppers, olive oil, lemon juice, dill, salt, and pepper in a large bowl, and stir until thoroughly mixed. Serve immediately or chill first.

Good for You

Sweet green peas have lots of starchy energy without any gluten, and I think they are one of the ultimate comfort foods. Try this salad for a happy lunch.

Tuna Twist

This tuna salad gets an update with tender pasta, crunchy cucumber, and capers.

6 ounces tuna, water-packed canned light tuna or flaked grilled tuna

1 cup cooked brown rice or quinoa pasta: twists, elbows, shells, penne, or whatever stubby shape you can find (preferably whole-grain)

$1/_2$ cup English ("seedless") cucumber, finely chopped

$1/_2$ cup shredded carrot

1 hardboiled egg, peeled and chopped

$1/_4$ cup capers, drained (from a jar)

1 tablespoon pimento, drained (from a jar)

1 tablespoon mayonnaise or plain yogurt

1 teaspoon dried or 1 tablespoon chopped fresh basil

8 large lettuce leaves

2 tomatoes, thinly sliced

> *Serves 4*

1. Combine tuna, rice or pasta, cucumber, carrot, egg, capers, pimento, mayonnaise or yogurt, and basil in a medium bowl. Mix thoroughly.

2. Arrange lettuce leaves on a large platter or four individual salad plates. Put a scoop of tuna salad on each lettuce leaf, and then surround with tomato slices. Serve immediately. You can eat this like a traditional salad, or roll lettuce leaves around the filling and eat it like a wrap.

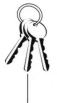

Good for You

Packed with protein and omega-3 fatty acids, tuna is an old stand-by, but choose the water-packed light (not albacore) variety for lower mercury content. Or make this recipe with leftovers from whenever you grill tuna steaks or filets. This is also a good way to use up leftover pasta.

Tropical Chicken Salad

Chicken, celery, and crunchy water chestnuts go tropical with added pineapple and tangerines.

Serves 4

2 cups cooked chicken, shredded

1 cup fresh or canned pineapple chunks

¹/₂ cup fresh tangerine or canned drained mandarin orange slices, halved

¹/₂ cup minced celery

¹/₄ cup diced water chestnuts, canned, drained

¹/₄ cup shredded coconut (optional—I know a lot of people don't like coconut, but I love it in this salad)

8 macadamia nuts, coarsely chopped

Juice from 1 fresh lime

¹/₄ teaspoon sea salt

Freshly ground black pepper

8 cups leafy greens

1. Combine chicken, pineapple, tangerine or orange slices, celery, water chestnuts, coconut, macadamia nuts, lime juice, salt, and pepper in a medium bowl and mix thoroughly. Serve piled on top of greens, on a platter or on individual salad plates. This also tastes good wrapped in a rice flour tortilla or tossed with cooked rice and a little wine vinegar.

Curried Broccoli Salad with Bacon

A classic broccoli salad with bacon and sunflower seeds tastes more exotic with spicy curry powder.

2 slices gluten-free bacon, cooked until crispy and drained (blot excess grease with a paper towel)

1 head broccoli, cut into bite-size florets

¹/₂ red onion, coarsely chopped and rinsed in a colander

¹/₂ cup sunflower seeds

¹/₄ cup raisins

1 tablespoon red wine vinegar

1 tablespoon apple cider vinegar

2 tablespoons mayonnaise

1 tablespoon milk

1 teaspoon curry powder

Serves 4

1. Combine bacon, broccoli, onion, sunflower seeds, raisins, and vinegars in a large bowl.

2. In a small bowl, combine mayonnaise, milk, and curry powder until ingredients are completely incorporated. Drizzle over salad, and toss to coat.

3. Let salad sit in the refrigerator for at least two hours or overnight. Serve cold.

Good for You

They say bacon makes everything better. It certainly makes everything saltier and fattier … but it sure tastes good. You only need a little bit in this recipe, for flavor. You can also use a soy-based vegetarian bacon like tempeh bacon, if you can find a gluten-free variety. Or leave bacon out entirely—it will still be good.

Personally, I think curry powder makes everything better, and this salad combines both flavors into an interesting and complex dish. Make this recipe a day ahead for the best flavor. If you don't like curry, substitute paprika (smoked Spanish paprika, a.k.a. *Pimentón*, makes an excellent alternative, if you can find it).

Soups

Warm, comforting, and nutrient-dense, soup will fill you up without adding a lot of unnecessary calories to your diet. Soup is also an excellent way to use up the produce in your refrigerator or take advantage of the very freshest vegetables in season. Try these savory soups and one sweet one, too, for light but satisfying fare.

Spicy Gazpacho

Like salsa in a soup bowl, this gazpacho is redolent with fresh tomatoes, juicy cucumbers, red bell peppers, and a dash of hot sauce for spice.

Serves 4

4 tomatoes, peeled, cored, finely chopped (save those juices!)

1 additional tomato, peeled, cored, and pureed to liquid in a blender

1 English ("seedless") cucumber, finely chopped

1 red bell pepper, cored, seeded, and finely chopped

$1/2$ red onion, finely chopped and rinsed in a colander

1 stalk celery, finely chopped

1 clove garlic, peeled and minced

1 tablespoon extra virgin olive oil

Juice from one fresh lemon

$1/2$ teaspoon sea salt

Freshly ground black pepper

Tabasco sauce or chipotle pepper sauce to taste (a couple of drops per person will make it zippy)

For garnish:

4 celery stalks with leaves

4 dill pickle spears

4 teaspoons chopped fresh cilantro

1. In a large bowl with a spout (I use an eight-cup glass measure), combine tomatoes, cucumber, bell pepper, onion, celery, garlic, olive oil, lemon juice, salt, and pepper. Refrigerate for at least two hours or overnight.

2. To serve, ladle soup into mugs. Add a spoon, a celery stalk, and a pickle spear to each mug. Sprinkle each with a teaspoon cilantro. Serve cold.

Good for You

I like this soup in the summer, served ice cold in mugs with a spoon, garnished with stalks of celery and pickle spears—like a Bloody Mary, but much better for you! Many gazpacho recipes contain a lot of vinegar, but I prefer just the lemon juice and a little olive oil. Add it back in if you like it, though. I won't be offended.

To peel tomatoes, dunk them via a slotted spoon or wire mesh strainer into boiling water for about ten seconds, then rinse in cold water. The skins should slip right off. Or, if you're feeling lazy, just leave the skins on. If they are chopped up well enough, it won't matter (unless you are fussy about such things).

French Onion Soup

Warm, savory, and full of flavor, this French Onion Soup gets a dash of sherry and doesn't need a slice of bread.

Serves 4

---

2 tablespoons olive oil, divided in half

4 yellow onions, peeled and thickly sliced, separated into rings

4 Portabella mushroom caps, about 4 inches in diameter, trimmed

1 tablespoon butter, melted

1 teaspoon ground cumin

1/4 teaspoon sea salt

1/2 teaspoon black pepper

1/2 cup dry sherry

2 teaspoons cornstarch dissolved in 2 tablespoons water

4 cups good-quality gluten-free canned beef broth (If you are really ambitious, use homemade beef stock. You can also substitute gluten-free vegetable broth.)

4 ounces shredded Gruyère or Swiss cheese (about one cup)

1. Preheat oven to 400°. Grease a roasting pan with 1 tablespoon olive oil. Arrange onions and mushroom caps in the pan. Combine remaining olive oil with melted butter, and drizzle mixture over mushrooms and onions. Sprinkle onions with cumin. Sprinkle onions and mushrooms with salt and pepper.

2. Roast onions and mushrooms for one hour or until deep golden brown and sizzling. Remove mushrooms to a separate plate and set aside. Put onions into a soup pot or Dutch oven, and set over medium-high heat on the stove.

3. Pour sherry into the hot roasting pan, and scrape off any vegetable bits. Pour and scrape entire mixture into the soup pot, over onions. While stirring, add cornstarch mixture. Then add beef broth, stirring constantly. As soon as soup starts to bubble, turn the heat to low and cover. Cook for 30 minutes or until soup starts to thicken.

4. Preheat the broiler. Put four oven-proof crocks or bowls on a heavy baking sheet. Ladle soup into crocks. Top each with a mushroom cap, and sprinkle cheese over each bowl. Broil for several minutes or until cheese is golden and bubbly. Serve immediately.

Good for You

Who says French onion soup has to contain bread? The French? Well, we're not in France, so I'm going to take a few liberties (my apologies to purists). I think a roasted portabella mushroom cap stands in perfectly well for that stale slice of bread and holds the cheese majestically on top of the soup. Roasting all the veggies first, instead of frying them, brings out a deep caramelized flavor. *Bon appétit!*

Tuscan-Style Beans & Greens Soup

A deeply comforting and nutritious dish filled with vegetables and hearty beans.

Serves 4

1 tablespoon olive oil

1 yellow onion, peeled and chopped

1 leek, trimmed and thinly sliced

1 stalk celery, trimmed and thinly sliced

1 red bell pepper, cored, seeded, and cut into thin strips

1 small zucchini, trimmed and diced

1 carrot, scrubbed and thinly sliced

4 cups chopped fresh kale

2 cloves garlic, peeled and minced

2 large tomatoes, cored and coarsely chopped

1 red potato, cut into small cubes

1 turnip or parsnip, trimmed and cut into small cubes

1 teaspoon dried or 1 tablespoon chopped fresh oregano

1 teaspoon dried or 1 tablespoon chopped fresh thyme

4 cups water

1 teaspoon sea salt

Freshly ground black pepper, to taste

Dash of red pepper flakes

2 cans white beans, drained and rinsed (*cannellini* or Great Northern beans)

4 slices gluten-free bread, toasted (optional)

Extra virgin olive oil and more black pepper, for garnish

1. In a large Dutch oven or soup pot, heat olive oil over medium-high heat. Add onions and leeks, and sauté until soft and just starting to brown, about 10 minutes. Add celery and sauté for an additional 3 minutes or so until celery gets soft. Add bell pepper, zucchini, and carrot. Sauté for 10 more minutes to fully soften and incorporate flavors. Add kale and garlic, and stir constantly until kale softens, about 5 minutes. Add tomatoes and stir for 3 more minutes.

2. Add potatoes, turnip or parsnip, oregano, thyme, and water. Stir once or twice to combine everything. Stop stirring. When soup just starts to bubble, stir in salt, black pepper,

red pepper flakes, and beans. Cover and allow to simmer for
2 hours. Keep an eye on it, stirring occasionally to prevent
vegetables from sticking to the bottom of the pan.

3. After soup cooks, you can either serve it or let it cool, put it in
the refrigerator, and reheat it tomorrow. When you do serve it
(now or tomorrow), tear optional toasted bread into pieces and
divide it between four bowls; then ladle soup over it. Or just
put soup into the bowls without bread. Drizzle each serving
with a little extra virgin olive oil and serve.

Good for You

My Italia-phile friend Richard calls this *ribollita*, Italian
for "cooked again." The recipe can be as varied as you
like—many Italian home cooks have their own versions. The
basic premise is a soup of greens, beans, and vegetables,
simmered for a long time, then reheated the next day. (That just
means it's even better the second day, but you can still eat it the
day you make it.) Use whatever vegetables you have, especially
winter vegetables. Richard says this soup should be ladled over
day-old bread. Since gluten-free bread tends to be stiffish, it will
work fine. Or just eat it without the bread. The beans provide
plenty of starch and fiber. This is also a great soup to make in
the crockpot if you are one of those crockpot people (like I am).

It might be tempting to just add all the vegetables at once, but
cooking them in stages, as indicated in this recipe, really does
give this soup its unique Italian flavor. There are times to be
creative and times to follow the recipe. In this case, follow the
recipe. You won't be sorry.

Spanish Chicken-and-Rice Soup

This hearty, smoky chicken soup with rice is a full meal on its own.

Serves 4

One whole chicken, cut into pieces (if you want to make this vegetarian, cut two pounds of drained extra-firm tofu into cubes, and use it as you would the chicken).

Sea salt

Freshly ground black pepper

1 tablespoon olive oil

1 large yellow onion, peeled and chopped

4 cloves garlic, peeled and thinly sliced

1 green bell pepper, cored, seeded, and cut into bite-size pieces

$^1/_2$ cup raw long-grain enriched white rice or brown rice

1 teaspoon smoked Spanish paprika (or regular paprika and dash of gluten-free chipotle sauce and/or liquid smoke), plus additional paprika for garnish

Pinch of saffron threads or turmeric

6 cups gluten-free chicken broth, homemade chicken stock, or gluten-free vegetable broth/stock

Hardboiled egg, sliced, for garnish (optional, but gives this soup a Spanish flair)

1. Season chicken pieces with salt and pepper. Heat olive oil in a large skillet over medium-high heat. Brown chicken pieces, remove them to a plate, and set aside.

2. Put onions in the pan, and sauté until golden, about 10 minutes. Add garlic and sauté for an additional 2 minutes. Add bell pepper, and sauté an additional 5 minutes. Add rice, paprika, and saffron. Sauté, stirring constantly, for about 3 minutes, thoroughly coating rice with oil and spices.

3. Add broth and return chicken pieces to the pot. Bring to a boil, lower the heat, and cover. Simmer for about 40 minutes or until rice is tender, stirring occasionally to prevent sticking (add water or additional broth if soup gets too thick).

4. To serve, ladle into bowls, and float a couple of hardboiled egg slices on top of each bowl. Sprinkle with additional paprika, and serve hot.

Good for You

This soup features my very favorite spice on earth—
Pimentón de la Vera, a.k.a. smoked Spanish paprika. If you
can't find it, just use regular paprika and (optionally) a dash
of liquid smoke or chipotle sauce (make sure it's gluten-
free). It won't be as good, but it will still give you the right idea.
This soup also contains that Spanish staple, saffron, notoriously
the most expensive spice in the world. But you can buy it in
very small amounts, in gourmet or ethnic stores. If you can't find
it, substitute turmeric. Again, not as good, but still good.

Harvest Pumpkin Soup

Garlic and cumin plus cinnamon and cloves give this pumpkin soup an interesting and seasonal complexity.

Serves 4

1 tablespoon olive oil

1 yellow onion, peeled and chopped

1 clove garlic, peeled and minced

$^1/_2$ teaspoon cumin

$^1/_4$ teaspoon cinnamon

Dash of ground cloves

$^1/_2$ teaspoon salt

Freshly ground black pepper, to taste

1 can pumpkin puree (*not* pumpkin pie mix)

1 can gluten-free chicken broth or gluten-free vegetable broth

4 teaspoons sour cream or plain yogurt, for garnish (optional)

1. Heat olive oil in a Dutch oven or soup pot. Add onion and sauté until golden, about 10 minutes. Add garlic, cumin, cinnamon, cloves, salt, and pepper. Sauté for 3 minutes.

2. Add pumpkin puree and broth. Combine thoroughly, then bring to a boil, stirring constantly. Reduce heat and simmer for 10 minutes. Serve hot, garnished with a pumpkin or squash flower (if you can find them) and a dollop of sour cream or plain yogurt.

Good for You

This spicy savory pumpkin soup makes a perfect Thanksgiving starter, but I like it all fall and winter long. It's also packed with antioxidants. And cinnamon! Plus, it's easy.

Orchard Fruit Soup with Vanilla Cream

Fresh juicy fruit makes the soup and creamy yogurt tops it off.

4 peaches, peeled, coarsely chopped (reserve juices)

4 pears, peeled, coarsely chopped (reserve juices)

8 plums, peeled, coarsely chopped (reserve juices)

Juice from one freshly squeezed lemon

1 cup apple cider or apple juice

$^1/_4$ cup plus 1 tablespoon honey or pure maple syrup

$^1/_2$ teaspoon cinnamon

$^1/_2$ cup vanilla yogurt or sour cream with $^1/_4$ teaspoon vanilla

Fresh blueberries or strawberry slices, for garnish

> *Serves 4*

1. Combine peaches, pears, plums, and all juices in a large bowl. Mash gently with a potato masher or the back of a wooden spoon until most larger chunks are broken down. (If you want the soup smoother, you can puree it in a blender, but I like it a little bit chunky).

2. Add cider or juice, $^1/_4$ cup honey or maple syrup, and cinnamon, and stir to combine. Chill for 1 hour (not much longer or it can start to turn brownish).

3. Meanwhile, make cream by combining yogurt or sour cream and vanilla with remaining tablespoon honey or maple syrup. Chill until ready to use.

4. Pour chilled soup into bowls or mugs and garnish with cream and blueberries or strawberry slices.

Entrées

Of course, you can always make a meal out of a big salad, a bowl of soup, and/or a collection of various side dishes, appetizers, or snacks. But this section focuses on the entrée, the heart of the meal—something that fills the center of your plate and makes you feel like you've really had dinner. Pair any of these meals with a salad, soup, and/or side dish from other sections in this mini cookbook, and you'll feel deliciously well fed.

Island Salmon with Mango-Lime Chutney

Crisp, moist broiled salmon gets exotic with spicy mango chutney on top.

For the chutney:

2 just-ripe mangoes, peeled and diced

2 cloves garlic, peeled and minced

$^1/_2$ red onion, peeled and finely chopped

1 small jalapeno pepper, seeded and minced

1 tablespoon fresh ginger root, peeled and minced

$^1/_2$ teaspoon sea salt

$^1/_2$ cup honey or pure maple syrup

$^1/_2$ cup white wine or white grape juice

$^1/_2$ cup cider vinegar

For the salmon:

1$^1/_2$ pound salmon filet

1 tablespoon olive oil

1 tablespoon ground cumin

$^1/_2$ teaspoon black pepper

$^1/_2$ teaspoon kosher salt

Dash of cayenne pepper

Serves 4

1. In a medium saucepan, combine mangoes, garlic, onion, pepper, ginger, and salt. Stir to combine. Add honey or maple syrup, wine or grape juice, and vinegar. Heat over medium-high until mixture just comes to a boil. Reduce heat and simmer for 20 minutes, stirring constantly. Remove from heat and allow to cool completely.

2. Preheat the broiler. Rinse salmon filet, and pat it dry with paper towels. Put salmon skin-side down on the broiler pan. In a small bowl, combine olive oil, cumin, black pepper, salt, and cayenne pepper. Rub this paste over salmon filet. Broil until done, about 15 minutes.

3. To serve, remove salmon to a plate. Cut into four portions, and serve with chutney. The Orange Cilantro Quinoa in the "Sides" section goes great with this, too.

Black Bean Quesadillas

Rich black beans, spicy chilies, smoky cumin, and low-fat mozzarella make these yummy quesadillas family-friendly.

Serves 4

1 can (15 ounces) black beans, drained and rinsed

1 can (4 ounces) green chilies, diced

½ teaspoon cumin

Freshly ground black pepper, to taste

1 cup cooked shredded chicken (optional)

8 corn tortillas

1 tablespoon canola oil

8 ounces (2 cups) shredded low-fat cheddar-jack cheese

Shredded lettuce, chopped tomatoes, sour cream, salsa, fresh corn for serving (optional)

1. In a medium saucepan over medium heat, combine beans, chilies, cumin, and pepper. Thin them with a little water, stirring and mashing, until hot (about 5 minutes).

2. Preheat oven to 400°. Brush or spray one side of four tortillas with oil, and put them on a large baking sheet. Top each tortilla with ¼ cup cheese. Divide bean mixture between four tortillas, and spread it over cheese, mashing it down so it comes almost to the edges of the tortilla. Top each with ¼ cup shredded chicken, if using. Top each with ¼ cup additional cheese and remaining tortillas. Press each top tortilla down gently, then brush or spray remaining oil on top of each quesadilla.

3. Bake until tortillas turn crispy on top, about 20 minutes (watch them to be sure they don't burn); then carefully flip each quesadilla and bake an additional 15 minutes or until entire quesadilla is crispy. Remove from the oven, and cool for about 5 minutes. Cut quesadillas into quarters with a pizza cutter or sharp knife. Serve with shredded lettuce, chopped tomatoes, sour cream, salsa, fresh corn, and/or Whipped Sweet Potatoes (see "Sides" section).

Good for You

The kids always breathe a sigh of relief when I say we're having quesadillas for dinner—because they know it will be good. Granted, one of my kids doesn't like the beans. So it's cheese only for him. But for the rest of us, this black-bean version, with or without chicken, is a favorite. I like to serve this with Whipped Sweet Potatoes (see "Sides" section). Sometimes I even spread them on top of the quesadilla, but everybody else in the family thinks that's weird.

Turkey Rice Pie

Homemade pot pie with a rice crust makes this warm, savory comfort-food entirely gluten-free.

Serves 4 (generously)

2 cups cooked rice (the stickier, the better, although brown rice is the most nutritious choice)

1 tablespoon white wine vinegar

1 teaspoon salt, divided in half

1¹/₂ teaspoons canola oil, divided

1 white onion, peeled and chopped

1 stalk celery, trimmed and minced

1 cup mushrooms, wiped clean and thinly sliced

¹/₂ cup green peas, fresh, frozen, or canned

1 carrot, shredded

1 teaspoon dried sage, plus a little extra for the top

Freshly ground black pepper to taste

1 cup dry white wine or gluten-free broth

¹/₄ cup cornstarch

¹/₂ cup water or gluten-free broth

2 cups cooked turkey, shredded or cut into bite-size chunks (also use chicken, pork, beef, or any other meat, or substitute cubes of drained tofu tossed with a little gluten-free tamari and briefly sautéed in canola oil)

1. Sprinkle vinegar and ¹/₂ teaspoon salt over rice, and mix to combine. Coat a pie plate (deep dish works best) with ¹/₂ teaspoon oil, and press rice into the pie plate and up the sides, shaping it into a crust by pressing it down with your hands or the back of a wooden spoon. Refrigerate until you're ready to use it.

2. Put remaining oil in a skillet over medium-high heat. Add onion and celery. Sauté until soft, about 5 minutes. Add mushrooms and sauté until soft, about 5 to 7 more minutes. Remove from the heat. Stir in peas and carrot. Sprinkle with sage, remaining salt, and pepper. Stir to combine. Remove everything from the pan and set aside in a bowl. Return the pan to the stove and deglaze with the wine or gluten-free broth, scraping to remove any bits of veggies.

3. Preheat the oven to 375°. In a small bowl, combine cornstarch and water or broth, stirring until cornstarch dissolves. Add this to the skillet and cook, stirring constantly, until the mixture thickens into gravy. Return all the vegetables and turkeys to the pan and stir to combine everything. Put turkey/veggie mixture into pie shell, and press it down with a spoon. Sprinkle with a little additional sage.

4. Bake pie for 40 minutes or until sizzling. Remove from the oven, and let it cool for 15 minutes. Cut into four to six wedges and serve. (All this needs on the side is a good salad.)

Good for You

This dinner "pie" uses a rice crust, making it a unique entrée that people seem to find very interesting. Plus, it tastes great and is a good way to use leftover rice. It works best with sticky short-grain rice (Tricia says preferably brown) like you would use to make sushi rolls, rather than the long-grain kind that doesn't really stick together. I've also made this with leftover rice from Chinese takeout. You can also vary the vegetables, as long as you keep the proportions about the same—approximately equal amounts of veggies and meat/tofu.

You can go a lot of different ways with this pie. I've thrown in a few leftover water chestnuts, some chopped kale instead of celery, leftover corn, some chopped tomatoes, black beans ... whatever you have around. Make it Asianish with chicken, water chestnuts, bok choy, celery, mushrooms, and gluten-free tamari instead of sage. Make it Mexican with corn, black beans, some salsa, and oregano or cilantro instead of the sage, then sprinkle a little cheese on the top. For the recipe as is, you can also add some Parmesan on top, but I usually just sprinkle on a little more sage. It's more pot-pieish without the cheese, which I find comforting.

Pork Chops and Applesauce

This old-school supper combines juicy pork with sweet apples and savory onions.

1 teaspoon canola oil

4 pork chops (with bones or boneless, but about 4 ounces of meat on each)

$\frac{1}{2}$ teaspoon salt

$\frac{1}{2}$ teaspoon paprika

1 apple, cored and thinly sliced

1 tablespoon brown sugar

1 teaspoon cinnamon

1 cup apple juice or cider

1 white onion, peeled and sliced

1 tablespoon cornstarch dissolved in 2 tablespoons water

$\frac{1}{2}$ cup milk

1. Preheat the oven to 350°. Put oil in a skillet, and heat on high. Sear pork chops for about a minute on each side. Put them in a large baking dish. Sprinkle with salt and paprika. (Reserve skillet for later—don't wash it yet.)

2. Spread apple slices evenly over pork chops. Sprinkle brown sugar and cinnamon over apples. Pour apple juice into the bottom of the pan (not over chops). Arrange onions around chops, bake for about 30 minutes, and remove from the oven.

3. Put pork chops with apples and onions on a serving plate, and cover loosely with foil. Scrape contents of the baking pan back into the skillet you used to sear chops. Heat on medium-high until just starting to bubble. Add cornstarch-water mixture and cook, stirring constantly, until gravy thickens, scraping browned bits from the bottom. Stir in milk. Remove from heat, pour gravy over pork chops, and serve with onions on the side. This recipe is good with roasted potatoes. You can roast potatoes and pork chops at the same time on different racks of the oven if you have the space.

Good for You _____

Remember that episode of *The Brady Bunch* where Peter tries to sound like Humphrey Bogart (or was it James Cagney) and repeats the dinner menu: "Pork chops and applesauce ..."? Whoops, am I dating myself? Anyway, it's a classic all-American dinner, but in this recipe, we combine the two elements into one to make the dish seem a little less "mod" and a little more classic. You can also substitute slices of drained, extra-firm tofu for the pork chops.

Nutty Basil Pasta

Crunchy nuts, healthy oil, and lots of fresh basil make this pasta into a sort of deconstructed pesto.

Serves 4

12 ounces gluten-free whole grain or enriched pasta

1 tablespoon extra virgin olive oil

1 clove garlic, finely minced

$^1/_2$ cup grated Parmesan cheese

$^1/_4$ teaspoon nutmeg

$^1/_3$ cup pine nuts

$^1/_3$ cup sliced almonds

$^1/_3$ cup walnuts

$^1/_2$ cup fresh basil, cut into fine shreds

1. Cook pasta according to package directions. Put it in a big bowl and toss with oil and garlic.

2. In a small bowl, combine cheese and nutmeg. Sprinkle over pasta, and toss to coat. Add pine nuts, almonds, and walnuts, and toss to combine. Stir in basil and serve immediately.

Sides and Snacks

Behind every great entrée is an even greater side dish! Okay, that might not really be true, but side dishes really can make the meal, highlighting and complementing the entrée. Or eat tapas-style, and make a meal of several side dishes. We've also added snacks to this section because a lot of side dishes can double as delicious snacks—not quite a meal, but satisfying.

Orange Cilantro Quinoa

Quinoa gets a citrusy zip with oranges and lemons.

1 teaspoon olive oil	**1 tablespoon orange zest**
¹/₂ yellow onion, minced	**Juice from one freshly squeezed lemon**
1 cup quinoa	
2 cups water	**¹/₂ cup chopped fresh cilantro leaves**
¹/₂ cup drained mandarin orange slices	**Salt and pepper to taste**
¹/₂ cup orange juice	**Chopped green onions for garnish**

> *Serves 4*

1. In a large skillet or soup pot with a lid, heat olive oil over medium-high heat. Sauté onion until translucent, about 10 minutes. Add quinoa and toss to coat. Add water. Stir for1 minute; then reduce heat to medium-low and cover. Simmer until all liquid is absorbed, about 15 minutes. If quinoa isn't tender, add a little more water.

2. Remove from heat, and stir in orange slices, orange juice, zest, lemon juice, and cilantro. Add salt and pepper to taste. Serve warm or cold (cover and keep in the refrigerator for up to one day), garnished with green onions.

Good for You

Quinoa is the ultimate grain—super nutritious with a unique texture and a nutty flavor. This tangy version goes great with fish or chicken. Serve leftovers cold the next day as a salad.

Whipped Sweet Potatoes

Mellow, rich sweet potatoes sweetened with applesauce and cinnamon could almost be a dessert.

Serves 4

4 medium-size sweet potatoes, peeled and quartered

¹/₄ cup milk

1 tablespoon butter or olive oil

¹/₄ teaspoon salt

³/₄ cup applesauce

Dash of cinnamon

1. Boil sweet potatoes until a fork inserts easily into them, about 20 minutes. Drain water. Put hot sweet potatoes into a mixing bowl. Add milk, butter or oil, and salt. Beat with an electric mixer or a wooden spoon until smooth.

2. In a small bowl, combine applesauce and cinnamon. Stir into potatoes and serve hot.

Green Onion Guacamole

Guacamole goes minimalist with just a little lemon, garlic, and green onion.

2 ripe avocadoes, preferably Hass

Juice from one fresh lemon

1 clove garlic, peeled and minced

4 green onions, coarsely chopped, including most of the greens

¼ cup chopped fresh cilantro

Serves 4

1. Peel, pit, and mash avocadoes.

2. Stir in lemon juice. Stir in garlic, onions, and cilantro. Serve immediately.

Good for You

Technically, an avocado may be a fruit, but I still call it my favorite vegetable. I make a lot of different kinds of guacamole, but this is one of my favorites. It's very simple and clean-tasting. I like to serve it with tortilla chips or on top of salad, but sometimes I just have a little as a side dish or condiment to the main meal.

Polenta with Marinara Mushroom Sauce

This herbed mushroom marinara tastes great ladled over crispy fried polenta.

Serves 4

2¼ cups water

1 teaspoon salt

1 cup quick-cooking polenta

1 tablespoon butter, divided

3 teaspoons olive oil, divided

1 clove garlic, minced

1 cup sliced mushrooms

1 15-ounce can crushed tomatoes

¼ cup chopped fresh basil or 1 tablespoon dried basil

1 tablespoon chopped fresh thyme or 1 teaspoon dried thyme

Salt and black pepper to taste

1. Bring water and salt to a boil in a large pot. Pour polenta into water in a stream so it doesn't stop boiling. Stir, lower the heat, and simmer, stirring constantly for 5 minutes. Remove from heat and stir in butter. Pour/spoon polenta into a loaf pan, and put it in the refrigerator to chill for about 30 minutes.

2. Meanwhile, heat 1 teaspoon olive oil over medium-high in a skillet. Add garlic and cook, stirring constantly, until just starting to turn color, about 5 minutes. Add mushrooms and sauté until they soften, about 10 minutes. Stir in crushed tomatoes, basil, and thyme. Simmer for about 30 minutes.

3. While sauce is simmering, preheat the oven to 400. Remove polenta, and turn it out onto a plate. Slice loaf and put slices on a baking sheet. Brush with remaining oil. Bake polenta for about 30 minutes, turning halfway through cooking time or until just starting to turn crispy and golden. Remove polenta to plates or a platter, and top with hot sauce. Serve immediately.

Good for You

I love this polenta recipe for a main course light meal, but it's also a delicious side dish, especially with pork or beef.

Roasted Potatoes with Peppers and Fennel

Potatoes roasted with vegetables and the anise-like fennel bulb give a basic side a French twist.

2 large or 8 small red potatoes

1 yellow onion, peeled and diced

1 green bell pepper, cored, seeded, and diced

1 red bell pepper, cored, seeded, and diced

1 fennel bulb, trimmed and very thinly sliced

1 tablespoon olive oil, divided

2 cloves garlic, minced

1 teaspoon kosher salt

1 tablespoon fresh or 1 teaspoon dried rosemary leaves

1 tablespoon fresh or 1 teaspoon dried thyme

Black pepper to taste

Red pepper flakes to taste

> *Serves 4*

1. Preheat the oven to 400°. Cut out any bad spots on potatoes, including "eyes," and cut into bite-size pieces. Put them in a large bowl.

2. Add onion, green and red peppers, and fennel. Drizzle with olive oil, and toss to coat everything. Spread vegetables on a large baking sheet with a rim. Sprinkle garlic, salt, rosemary, thyme, pepper, and red pepper flakes evenly over vegetables.

3. Bake for about 40 minutes or until potatoes are fork-tender, stirring every 15 or 20 minutes so vegetables don't stick. Serve hot. Leftovers are good the next day, served cold and tossed with a little of your favorite salad dressing.

 Good for You

I like to make these roasted potatoes when fennel comes into season. If you don't like the licorice-y taste of fennel (lots of people don't), substitute carrots or leeks.

Tahini Dip with Crudité

Like hummus without the garbanzo beans, this tahini combines rich sesame paste with zesty lemon and flavorful garlic.

Serves 4

³/₄ cup tahini (sesame paste)

¹/₄ cup water or milk

Juice and zest from 1 fresh lemon

1 tablespoon olive oil

1 garlic clove, peeled and minced

¹/₂ teaspoon salt

Paprika for garnish

Cut-up raw vegetables for serving (carrot sticks, bell pepper strips, cucumber spears, cherry tomatoes, broccoli and cauliflower florets, etc.)

1. Combine tahini, water, lemon juice and zest, oil, garlic, and salt in a medium serving bowl. Sprinkle paprika on top. Serve with raw veggies.

Good for You

With a substantial entrée, sometimes the only side dish I have on the table is a bunch of cut-up raw veggies and a really good dip. This tahini dip is one of my favorites.

Coconut Rice

Sweet creamy coconut milk adds rich flavor to butter-scented basmati rice.

³/₄ cup basmati rice

¹/₂ cup coconut milk

¹/₂ cup water

1 teaspoon lemon zest

¹/₂ teaspoon ground turmeric

¹/₂ teaspoon red pepper flakes (optional)

¹/₂-inch piece of fresh ginger, peeled (don't chop it up)

1 bay leaf

¹/₂ teaspoon salt

¹/₄ cup chopped fresh cilantro

¹/₄ cup sliced almonds

Serves 4

1. Combine rice, coconut milk, water, lemon zest, turmeric, pepper flakes, ginger, and bay leaf in a medium saucepan. Bring to a boil. Stir in salt. Lower heat and cover. Simmer until rice absorbs all liquid, about 20 minutes.

2. Remove and discard bay leaf and ginger. Stir in cilantro and almonds. Serve immediately.

Good for You

This exotic dish tastes great with fish, or go sweet and serve it with fresh pineapple.

Nacho Art

Nachos with anything *you* like, for a change—from olives and peppers to peas, beans, and corn!

Serves 4

8 corn tortillas, cut into quarters and baked in the oven until crisp

Toppings, such as:

Sliced olives

Diced tomatoes

Bell pepper strips

Shredded or sliced carrots

Pickle slices

Green peas

Corn

Salsa

Ketchup

Sour cream

Shredded low-fat cheese

1. Divide tortilla wedges between four plates. Sprinkle each with a little shredded cheese, and heat in the microwave to melt cheese slightly.

2. Let each person decorate his nachos as desired. Encourage creativity and more vegetables. Microwave individual servings to heat toppings, if desired.

Good for You

Isn't food more fun if it's *pretty?* Kids love making these do-it-yourself, colorful and creative nachos, and if they make them themselves, they are a lot more likely to eat them. (At least, theoretically!)

Desserts

Dessert certainly isn't a necessary part of a meal, and probably shouldn't follow every meal or even be a part of every day. Desserts are special treats for every now and then, unless you count a delicious, sweet, juicy piece of fruit as dessert, which, nutrition-wise, is an excellent idea.

In this section, you find lots of ideas for delicious gluten-free desserts—most of them made with fruit and relatively low in calories and fat but high in pleasure. Remember, dessert can be good for you even while it makes your life a little sweeter.

Sweet-Tart Crisp

Tart apples, crispy cereal, and sweet brown sugar flavor this fall dessert.

4 tart apples, like Granny Smith	**¹/₄ cup gluten-free crisp rice cereal**	*Serves 4*
Juice from one fresh lemon	**¹/₄ cup brown sugar**	
1 tablespoon butter, softened	**¹/₂ teaspoon cinnamon**	

1. Preheat the oven to 400°. Peel, core, and slice apples. Put them in a bowl and toss with lemon juice. Spread apples in the bottom of a pie plate.

2. In a small bowl, combine butter, rice cereal, brown sugar, and cinnamon. Mix with a fork until combined. Sprinkle mixture over apples. Bake until top gets crispy and golden, about 30 minutes. Serve warm with or without a dollop of vanilla ice cream.

Good for You

The best time to make apple crisp is in the fall when apples are peaking. Take the family out to a you-pick orchard and gather your own!

Tropical Fruit Salad

Favorites like oranges and bananas team up with more exotic fruits like mangoes and pomegranate seeds.

> **Serves 4**

1 orange, peeled and sectioned, cut into bite-size chunks

1 mango, peeled and cut into cubes

1 pineapple, peeled, cored, and cut into cubes

2 bananas, peeled and sliced

Seeds from one pomegranate

Juice from one lemon

Juice from one lime

Coconut shreds and/or fresh mint leaves for garnish

1. Combine orange, mango, pineapple, and banana pieces with pomegranate seeds. Drizzle with lemon and lime juice. Toss to coat. Garnish with coconut shreds and/or mint leaves. If you like it sweeter, sprinkle with a little sugar. (I prefer it without.)

Good for You

It takes a little time to peel, seed, pit, and chop these exotic fruits for Tropical Fruit Salad, but the combination is worth the effort.

Peachy Parfait

Layers of yogurt cushion tender chunks of ripe juicy peaches.

2 cups low or nonfat vanilla, lemon, or peach yogurt

1/4 teaspoon cinnamon, plus some for garnish

Dash of nutmeg

4 ripe peaches, pitted and cut into bite-size chunks

Juice from one fresh lemon

Serves 4

1. Combine yogurt with cinnamon and nutmeg in a small bowl. In another bowl, toss peach chunks with lemon juice.

2. In each of four tall wine or champagne glasses, layer spoonfuls of yogurt with spoonfuls of peach chunks. Begin and end with yogurt. Garnish with an additional dash of cinnamon.

Chocolate Whisper

These light, cocoa-flavored meringue cookies practically melt in your mouth.

2 egg whites at room temperature

1/4 teaspoon cream of tartar

1/4 cup superfine sugar

1 teaspoon vanilla

2 tablespoons cocoa powder

Makes 24 cookies

1. Preheat the oven to 350°. In a clean dry bowl, beat egg whites and cream of tartar with a wire whisk until soft peaks form. Continue beating as you add sugar, 1 tablespoon at a time, then vanilla, then cocoa powder, one tablespoon at a time, until stiff peaks form.

2. Spray a baking sheet with gluten-free cooking spray, or rub it lightly with oil. Drop heaping teaspoons of meringue onto the cookie sheet, or use a pastry tube to make swirly designs. Bake for about 15 minutes or until firm on top. Store in an airtight container … if you have any left.

Banana Popsicle

Who needs the ice cream truck when you've got creamy frozen bananas dipped in chocolate syrup?

Serves 4

4 bananas

4 popsicle sticks

¹/₂ cup gluten-free chocolate syrup (the stuff you use to make chocolate milk, like Hershey's)

1. Put a sheet of waxed paper or parchment paper on a baking sheet or shallow casserole that will fit in your freezer. Spray it with gluten-free cooking spray, or lightly rub it with oil.

2. Peel bananas, and stick a popsicle stick into one end of each. Pour chocolate syrup on a plate with a shallow edge. Roll each banana in chocolate to coat lightly, then put it on the baking sheet. Freeze until firm, about 2 hours or overnight.

Variation: After dipping bananas in chocolate syrup, roll them in gluten-free rice cereal for a healthy version of the old-fashioned drumstick.

Another variation: Melt ¹/₂ cup peanut butter with or without chocolate syrup, and dip bananas into warm peanut butter before it firms up again. Freeze as directed.

Good for You

Kids love this classic snack (I remember my mom making these when I was a kid), but grown-ups shouldn't let the kids have all the fun. Make a banana popsicle for everybody!

Maple Poached Pears with Nutmeg

Juicy soft pears flavored with brandy, maple, and nutmeg make an easy and elegant dessert.

1 750 ml. bottle flavorful white wine, like Chardonnay or Riesling

¹/₂ cup brandy or almond or orange liqueur

Juice from one fresh lemon

Juice from one fresh orange

¹/₂ cup real maple syrup

¹/₄ teaspoon nutmeg

4 firm ripe pears (soft ones will fall apart—Bosc or firm Anjou pears work well)

Serves 4

1. Combine wine, brandy or liqueur, lemon juice, orange juice, maple syrup, and nutmeg in a medium saucepan. Heat over medium-high until mixture begins to boil.

2. Meanwhile, carefully cut bottoms off pears so they will sit flat. Peel them, then carefully cut out cores from base without disturbing flesh. If you can, leave stems on. Brush or drizzle them with lemon juice.

3. Lower the heat to medium and gently lower pears into the liquid. Cover the pan, and cook them for about 20 minutes. The pears should be tender but not mushy or falling apart. Lift pears out carefully, and set them upright on plates. Cover loosely with plastic wrap and put them in the refrigerator.

4. Turn the heat to medium-high and continue to cook sauce until it is reduced by about half, about 30 minutes. Stir often. Spoon sauce around each pear and serve, or chill sauce, covered in the refrigerator, for up to 2 hours, and then serve.

Warm Applesauce Sundae

Warm cinnamon-flavored applesauce stands in for syrupy sundae sauce over frozen vanilla yogurt.

Serves 4

2 cups natural (unsweetened) applesauce

1 teaspoon cinnamon

2 cups low-fat frozen vanilla yogurt

4 tablespoons chopped pecans

1. Combine applesauce and cinnamon in a small saucepan. Heat over medium heat until warm, about 5 minutes. Stir often.

2. Put $1/2$-cup scoops of yogurt into each of four bowls. Pour $1/2$ cup warm applesauce over each scoop. Garnish each with one tablespoon pecans. Serve immediately.

Chocolate Chip Chow

Sweet chocolate with crunchy nuts and chewy dried fruit provide concentrated (and delicious) energy.

Serves 4

$1/2$ cup semi-sweet or bitter-sweet chocolate chips

$1/2$ cup sliced almonds

$1/2$ cup dried cherries or raisins

$1/2$ cup shredded coconut or dried banana chips or go crazy—use both! Or substitute something else like sunflower seeds or gluten-free cold cereal or dried apricots or anything else you like)

1. Mix chocolate chips, almonds, cherries, coconut, and anything else you like together. Eat.

Good for You

This is the perfect midafternoon pick-me-up snack when your sweet tooth is calling your name. Need I say more? Okay, I'll say more: this is also good stirred into yogurt or sprinkled on top of ice cream.

Fruit Kebobs with Yogurt Cream

Peaches, pears, apples, and oranges get skewered and dipped in creamy honey-sweetened yogurt.

1 cup plain low or nonfat yogurt

1 tablespoon honey

1 tablespoon orange juice

1 peach

1 pear

1 apple

1 orange

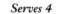
Serves 4

1. Combine yogurt, honey, and orange juice in a small bowl. Stir until smooth. Divide into four small bowls.

2. Core and cut peach, pear, and apple into bite-size chunks. Peel and section orange.

3. On 4 skewers, alternate chunks of peach, pear, apple, and orange. Serve with yogurt cream on the side.

Good for You

These assemble in minutes and make a fun way to eat fruit without having it drip down your chin.

Just a Trifle

Tender gluten-free cake chunks layered with strawberries, pudding, and cream make a beautiful dessert.

Serves 4

2 cups vanilla, tapioca, or butterscotch pudding made with low-fat milk (check the label to make sure the pudding is gluten-free—many instant puddings are okay because they are made with cornstarch)

2 cups bite-size chunks of gluten-free cake, made from a mix (your favorite flavor)

2 cups fresh strawberries, sliced

A little whipped cream for garnish

4 whole strawberries for garnish

In a tall glass bowl or trifle bowl, make layers of pudding, cake, strawberries, more pudding, more cake, more strawberries, and end with pudding. Garnish with a little whipped topping and whole strawberries. Serve by scooping it out into glass bowls.

Good for You

Is trifle old-fashioned? Do you care? I think this makes a very pretty dessert, especially when company comes over. This uses mostly packaged ingredients, so don't make it very often. It's got a lot of sugar, but it's easy. This is also a *great* solution when your homemade gluten-free cake falls apart and you need to serve dessert! Nobody will know it wasn't supposed to be a trifle in the first place.

Index

Equal, 73
explaining gluten-free diet to friends, 36

F

fajitas, 179
FALCPA (Food Allergen Labeling and Consumer Protection Act), 16
family/friends
  meetings with, 32
  misconceptions, 138-139
  personal challenges, 139-140
  refusing testing, 140-141
farina, 91
fast food, 194-195
fava beans, 73
FDA (Food and Drug Administration), 44-45
  food label rules, 44
  Gluten-Free Labeling Proposed Rule website, 102
  website, 23, 45
fiber, 212-213
finding
  gluten-free foods, 33-34
  gluten-free packaged foods, 117
  restaurants, 192-194
First Watch, 198
fish, 73
flavorings, 91
flaxseed, 73, 213
Flexible Sauce recipe, 169
flour, 91
  bread, 90
  brown rice, 69
  gluten-free, 91
  glutinous rice, 74
  unbleached, 96
  whole-wheat, 97
folate, 213

Food Allergen Labeling and Consumer Protection Act (FALCPA), 16
Food Allergy Kitchen group, 145
Food and Drug Administration. *See* FDA
Food and Wine, 152
foods
  additives, 51
  allergens. *See* allergens
  containing gluten. *See also* hidden gluten
    alphabetical listing of, 88-98
    baked goods, 16-18
    beer, 22, 89, 128-131
    beverages, 111
    blue cheese, 60
    breads, 16-18
    canned/boxed/bottled foods, 24-25, 107
    cereals/grains, 18-20
    condiments, 24
    dry foods, 108-109
    frozen foods, 25-26, 106
    ingredients lists, 23
    meats, 26
    snack foods, 24, 110
    soups, 25
    sweets, 20-21
    vegetarian, 23
  gluten-free
    beverages, 112
    canned/jarred/bottled foods, 107-108
    dry packaged foods, 110
    finding, 33-34
    frozen foods, 106-107
    labeling requirements, 55
    list of, 67-84, 115-117
    packaged. *See* packaged foods, gluten-free
    snack foods, 111

labels
  additives, 51
  allergens, 48
  anatomy, 44
  CONTAINS statements, 48
  FALCPA, 45
  FDA rules, 44
  gluten-free labeling, 45, 55
  ingredients lists, 45-47
  "manufactured in a facility that contains" statements, 49
  processed foods, 102-104
  wheat sources, 49-51
  processed/packaged. *See* processed foods; packaged foods
  pyramid website, 216
formal functions, 204-205
French toast, 91
FritoLay, Products Not Containing Gluten website, 110
frozen foods
  probably containing gluten, 25-26, 106
  probably gluten-free, 106-107
frozen yogurt, 73
fruit, 73, 214
  citrus, 70
  dried, 72
  juice, 74
  shopping list, 186

G

garbanzo beans, 74
Gardenburger, 122
Garlic Bread, 183
garro, 91
gastrointestinal symptoms, 7